Travel Therapy: Around the World in Search of Happiness

Stuart Katz

3rd Coast Books, LLC
19790 Hwy. 105 W. Ste. 1318
Montgomery, Texas 77356

Copyright © 2023 by Stuart Katz
Published by 3rd Coast Books, 2023

All Rights Reserved.
No part of this book may be reproduced or transmitted in any form or by any means, electronic or mechanical. This includes photocopying or recording by any information storage or retrieval system, without written permission from the publisher, except for brief quotations embodied in critical reviews.

3rd Coast Books, LLC
19790 Hwy. 105 W. Ste. 1318
Montgomery, TX 77356

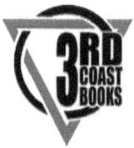

www.3rdCoastBooks.com

ISBNs
Hardcover – Color 978-1-946743-67-1
Hardcover – B&W 978-1-946743-66-4
Paperback – 978-1-946743-71-8
eBook/ePub – 978-1-946743-68-8

Project Coordinator - Ian W. Gorman, Associate Publisher
Editor - Ian W. Gorman
Cover Artist - Urška Charney
Layout - Urška Charney

Library of Congress Control Number: 2023912643

There is a crack in everything, that's how the light gets in.

— **Leonard Cohen**

TESTIMONIALS

"Your present mindset does not determine where you will go. It only tells you that this is the place you are starting from. If you stay here, it is likely that not too many things will change or when they do, will change slowly. That is because we mostly do the same thing over and over again. It is our nature. Oliver Wendell Holmes said that: 'A mind that is stretched by a new experience can never go back to its old dimensions.' In *Travel Therapy*, Stuart Katz takes us through his life journey, and how he, like all of us, is shaped by his upbringing and relationships with those closest to him. The stories of early childhood are sprinkled with earnest mirth and will bring a genuine smile to those who've been there. If this book were just about childhood, relationships, and faith, it would certainly be interesting but perhaps not of interest to as many. What makes this book stand out is just how profoundly Stuart's extensive travels throughout the world shape his worldview and impact his overall sense of self. Although his deep faith is resonant throughout the book, his views on so many 'certainties' change as he recognizes the aspirations of our fellow planetary travelers, and in so doing, recognizes his own yearning. We see that the best place on Earth is the Earth itself. The best people on Earth are the people themselves, and travel is the best way to kickstart a path to inevitable and healing growth."

— **Blaise Aguirre, MD**
Founding Medical Director, 3East DBT Continuum
The Michael Hollander, PhD, Endowed Director
Assistant Professor in Psychiatry
Harvard Medical School Department of Psychiatry

"Stuart's journey is an inspiration and a lesson in building resilience. Recovery is possible!"

— **Brian Cuban**
Author, *The Ambulance Chaser*

"Stuart Katz's darkest days have made him stronger. In his travel-themed memoir, Stuart shows us what it's like to struggle with mental health and how to triumph, in big and small ways, by leaning in and not away from the struggles. Stuart shares his enormous heart and his extensive travels with grace, humor, and refreshing vulnerability. What a mensch (true story)!"

— **Joshua Rivedal**
Author, *Mental Health Educator*, Standup Comic

"I've known and admired Stuart Katz for years, and I'm delighted to finally read his story in this excellent book. *Travel Therapy* combines travel memoir with a mental health journey. It also includes the stories of Stuart's extensive travel as a volunteer assisting in crisis areas and his exploration of Jewish communities across the globe, as he works towards visiting 100 countries, all the while in search of how to heal himself. Witty, self-deprecating, and heartfelt, this is a must-read for anyone interested in travel, Judaism, and the lifelong journey towards psychological wellbeing."

— **Rabbi Shmuley Boteach**
Rabbi, Author, Speaker, Television Host

"I've had the great honor of knowing Stuart Katz for many years, and he is a winner in every way. This book gives us not only tips for travel but tips for life. It also shows us how to turn challenges into springboards, not only for ourselves but for the people around us. Stuart is a perfect example of this. He's taken his challenges and not only used them to learn how to better take care of himself and his loved ones—he's dedicated his life to helping strangers in need. To me, that is the definition of a winner!"

— **Tamir Goodman**
"The Jewish Jordan"
Author, *The Jewish Jordan's Triple Threat: Physical, Mental, and Spiritual Lessons from the Court*

"Stuart Katz's captivating memoir delves into the transformative power of travel and service, and their profound impact on mental health. In this remarkable book, Katz fearlessly shares his own experiences in grappling with mental health challenges, and many of his realizations that came later in life, emerging from those personal battles. His candid and humorous storytelling draws readers into his world, allowing them to relate and intimately understand the impact that travel and service can have on one's healing journey."

— **Eric Kussin**
Founder/CEO, #SameHere Global Mental Health Movement

"Stuart really opens up about the nuances of your mindset when you are continuously maintaining your mental health. The guilt, the nitpicking you do to yourself, the constant need to do more and be more. Stuart Katz's take on mental health struggles and maintenance really speaks to the vulnerability we all have in a very easy to understand, conversational approach. Stuart's story is very relatable to anyone who has struggles. I believe that everyone can gain a lot of new insights and clarity into the battle to find yourself, a process we are all undertaking, one way or another."

— **Reggie Walker**
Former NFL Football Player

"Stuart Katz is a remarkable writer yet an even more remarkable human being. His vulnerability and openness when dealing with such complex issues will save many lives. I'm grateful to call Stuart my friend and to truly endorse this book as a must-read for anyone, but especially those dealing with mental health challenges: themselves, with their family or their friends."

— **Asher Gottesman**
Mental Health Professional
Founder, Transcend Recovery Community and Heights Treatment

"One of the most compelling aspects of *Travel Therapy* is how Stuart intertwines his personal growth as a Jew with his broader journey as a human being. He reflects on how his experiences abroad, aiding those in their darkest hours, ultimately shaped him into a better Jew and a better person. This nuanced exploration of spirituality and self-discovery adds a profound layer to the narrative, resonating with readers from all walks of life."

— **Michael Sweetney**
Former NBA Basketball Player
Assistant Coach, Yeshiva University Men's Basketball

"What sets *Travel Therapy* apart is Katz's unique ability to intertwine his personal narrative with a larger tapestry of universal truths. As readers accompany him on his journey, they are confronted with the undeniable reality that healing and happiness often lie in our service to others. Katz's unwavering dedication to making a positive impact on the lives of those he encounters serves as an inspiring testament to the remarkable resilience of the human spirit."

— **Zak Williams**
Mental Health Advocate & Entrepreneur

"I am thrilled by *Travel Therapy*, an extraordinary account of friendship that transcends boundaries, prejudice, and conflict. As a Syrian refugee who found solace and compassion in the most unexpected of places, this book resonated deeply with me.

"Within these pages, the story of an unlikely bond unfolds between me, a Syrian refugee, and an Israeli, my dear friend and brother, Stuart Katz. Our friendship serves as a powerful testament to the transformative power of genuine human connection, regardless of nationality, religion, race, or political beliefs. Our journey of mutual learning and support offers a profound example of what true friendship can be and an understanding that mental illness and mental well-being knows of no barriers.

"Through our shared experiences, the two of us continue to learn from one another, challenge preconceived notions, and break down the walls that historically divided our people. Our commitment to understanding, empathy, and compassion sets a remarkable example for us all, demonstrating that friendship can transcend even the most entrenched conflicts.

"Stuart beautifully captures the essence of resilience, hope, and the capacity for change that lies within each of us. It is a testament to the potential for personal growth and transformation that can emerge from the unlikeliest of circumstances.

"I highly recommend *Travel Therapy* to anyone seeking inspiration, enlightenment, and a renewed faith in the power of friendship. It serves as a timely reminder that humanity's greatest strength lies in our ability to connect, empathize, and stand together, regardless of our differences.

"May this book serve as a beacon of hope, fostering greater understanding and encouraging us all to build bridges, rather than fences. Let us together continue to embrace the spirit of compassion and friendship, and work towards a world where unity and harmony prevail.

"In a world often characterized by division and conflict, *Travel Therapy* offers a much-needed message of hope, reminding us that friendship can indeed transcend all barriers and strong mental health is possible for all. It is a testament to the power of human connection and a true inspiration for us all."

— **Gassen Alhoro**
Syrian Refugee now living in Germany

To Carol, this book is dedicated to you, my unwavering partner and companion throughout our incredible journey, spanning 37 years and over 50 countries. Your love, support, and presence have been my anchor as we've ventured to every corner of the globe.

CONTENTS

Foreword i
1 | Come Fly with Me 1
2 | Almost Dying Will Do That to You................................... 5
3 | A True International: My Life as a Panamanian 11
    American Israeli Jewish Citizen of the World
4 | My Partner in the Journey of Life................................ 21
5 | All My Honeymoons.. 27
6 | TAL Tours: How to Run a Travel Agency 35
7 | The $100,000 Fuel Bill: How to Run an Airline.................... 43
8 | The Morally Questionable Misadventures of Travel Clients 49
9 | Where Does a Traveler Call Home? 55
10 | Back Home as a Foreigner 69
11 | A Trip with Each Child 77
12 | Travel for Volunteer Work 123
13 | Transformational Travel is a Thing............................ 135
14 | Travel for Disaster Relief Work 145
15 | In Search of the Happiest Place on Earth..................... 157
16 | The Me Project: Investing in My Own Mental Health 167
17 | Addicted to Helping Others: Travels to Aid Refugees 173
18 | Therapy is a Journey.. 189
Epilogue 197
Acknowledgments 199
About the Author... 201

FOREWORD

I can't change the direction of the wind, but I can adjust my sails to always reach my destination.

— Jimmy Dean

I jumped.

I remember that day like it was yesterday, although it's been over two decades now. It was a bleak and desolate morning, the kind that wraps you in a heavy blanket of sadness. I was just nineteen years old, struggling with a darkness that seemed impossible to escape. My name is Kevin Hines, and this is the story of how my life changed from an absolute determination to end it, to a fierce will to live and to help others who feel as hopeless as I did. To tell them that suicide is not the answer.

I'd been suffering from epilepsy since childhood. When I weaned off the anti-seizure medication, aged sixteen, I thought my troubles were over. Turns out it was just the next chapter. I began to experience symptoms of bipolar disorder. Life felt empty, with no hope on the horizon. When my drama teacher died by suicide, I was devastated, but also saw this as a way out of my misery.

On September 25, 2000 — a Monday — I climbed aboard a bus and got off at the Golden Gate Bridge. This is suicide central: from 1937 to 2012, an estimated 1,400 people took their own lives by leaping off the bridge. The numbers are staggering. In 2013 alone, 118 potential suicides were standing on the bridge, ready to jump, but were talked down. That same year, thirty-four people tried to kill themselves but survived the attempt.

It's a long way down. 245 feet, a four-second fall. Most are killed by the impact, as your body hits the water at up to 75 - 80 miles per hour, at 15,000 pounds of pressure. You near the speed of terminal velocity. Then there are the twin dangers of drowning and hypothermia. There's a crisis counseling sign that reads "There is hope" on the bridge, but it's not enough. It wasn't for me.

As I stood on the edge of the Golden Gate Bridge, looking down at the churning waters below, my mind was consumed by a swirling storm of pain and despair. Thoughts of hopelessness echoed through my head, drowning out any glimmer of reason or clarity. Tears streamed down my face.

In that moment, I felt so alone, as if there was no one in the world who could understand the depth of my anguish. I felt trapped, suffocated by the weight of my own emotions. The voices in my head grew louder, telling me that there was only one way to escape the torment I was experiencing.

The voices inside my head had been telling me to die for months. They told me to throw myself off. Right. Now.

I jumped.

But the moment I did, I had instantaneous regret. My body was in freefall, and I suddenly was certain that I didn't want it to be. That I wanted to live. I somehow had enough of my wits about me to twist my body around, so I was no longer plummeting headfirst, but instead feet first. My legs split the water open like a mouth. The water was so cold as it swallowed me. I became submerged seventy feet beneath the surface of the water.

I somehow made my way to the circle of water above me, bobbing along the waves. I was shaking and stunned. Soon thereafter, I felt something bump against my leg. I looked down. What was it? I thought it was a shark, ready to sink its razor teeth into me at any moment. I couldn't believe it, my mind running blank.

I would learn later it was, in fact, a sea lion that stayed with me, helping keep me buoyant, until the Coast Guard arrived and hauled me out of the water. It's the most miraculous thing I've ever heard of.

Since that day, I have dedicated my life to spreading awareness about mental health, brain health, and suicide prevention. It was the turning point that set me on a path of healing and recovery. It showed me that, even in the depths of despair, there is always a glimmer of hope, a reason to keep fighting.

I've become an advocate, sharing my story with others who may be walking the same treacherous path I once walked. I want everyone to know that there is help available, that you are not alone, and that there is always hope.

Every day is still a struggle, but I've learned to find strength in my vulnerability and to reach out for support when I need it. I've come to understand that my story is not defined by my suicide attempt, but by the resilience and determination I've discovered in its aftermath.

So, if you find yourself standing on that edge, ready to take that final step, I implore you to pause, to reach out, and to hold on. There are people who care, who will listen, and who will walk beside you on the journey to healing. Remember, even in the darkest of moments, there is always hope.

All this brings me to what I love about this book. It's close to my heart and will be close to the hearts and minds of anyone who is on a mental health journey. That means everyone, really. Whether the issues one faces in the endless wrestling match with one's own mind are devastating or incidental inconveniences or anything in between, there's not a person alive who does not have moments of struggle. It's part of what makes us human. Alas, more severe and even potentially life-threatening issues affect so much of the world's population that, even if you don't feel the struggle yourself, chances are you've got a friend or family member who is swimming against the current of their own feelings and thoughts.

Books like this one can help. In *Travel Therapy*, Stuart Katz writes like a sympathetic friend, a charming, funny travel companion, but also someone selfless enough to open his own story up to the world, and to show how a life dedicated to helping others is a life well-lived.

Travel Therapy combines a fun travel memoir with three other elements: an exploration of Judaism across the globe, a look at how volunteering in crisis zones elevates the volunteer as much as it helps those in the depths of crisis, and how mental wellbeing is inevitably a metaphorical journey, as much as world travel is a literal one. Stuart's voice is immediately present — you can feel him throughout the text, his prose very much like his conversation. He's a copilot on this journey of life, someone you want to spend time with.

Stuart's stated goal with this book is to save at least one life. I'm sure he will, and far more than that. You've already completed half the battle by picking up this book. Read it and you will feel less alone. You will feel better.

Stuart is a survivor of depression, and he tells his story, and that of his family, with compassion, introspection, wisdom, and humor. His approach to dealing with mental illness has been to look globally. He travels the world, both as a warm-hearted volunteer in crisis zones and as a tourist truly and deeply interested in the experience of locals and international cultures. What can we learn from the way other nations deal with mental illness, and how can travel itself be a form of therapy?

You're in for a rewarding ride.

— **Kevin Hines**
Author, Storyteller, Filmmaker, and Brain Health Advocate

Chapter 1

Come Fly with Me

My dark days made me strong. Or maybe I already was strong, and they made me prove it.

— Emery Lord

Guilt is my copilot. I'm a guilt-fueled overachiever. I once couldn't remember if I'd paid the bar bill at a South Korean hotel — I probably did, but I got out of there in a hurry when I realized that the nice young woman eagerly chatting with me was actually (oops!) a prostitute — and I *still* feel guilty about it. (Note to self: maybe I should send an anonymous payment to the hotel for the price of a Diet Dr. Pepper, so I can sleep better at night). I'm home in Israel now, but I'm out of the country about 80% of the time. Nobody would know this — I'm sending messages every day. If you write to me and I don't write back, I'm either on an airplane or dead (or you just need to wait a bit, as I'm too cheap to pay for Wi-Fi). But I feel that, if I'm not physically present, I'm not doing the job right.

I feel tremendous guilt when I feel I'm not doing what should be done. I don't accept guilt from others, but I bear it myself. This is a hand-me-down from my family. I was the oldest child, and the oldest grandchild, on both sides. I didn't have a real childhood because I was made an adult from infancy. I feel that I must be the adult in the room, regardless of what I'm doing or how many other adults are there. I'm always multitasking. I'm obsessed with walking: I'm always wearing my Fitbit and I almost always take the stairs.

My brain wants to cover many fields at once, too. Even as I write this, I'm on call on a suicide prevention hotline, stopping frequently to assist others in need. I spent — or maybe I should say endured — ten years as president of various synagogues. I regularly fly around the world to places where people are in need: to Greece to help Syrian refugees, to Nepal to help after an earthquake, to post-typhoon Philippines, to hurricane-ripped New York, to work with the poor throughout Latin America and the Caribbean, to assist refugees from Ukraine. Smell a disaster and you can probably catch a whiff of well-meaning Stuart in the breeze. It's fair to say that I'm addicted to helping people.

This is a fine trait for a parent, for the head of an airline, for the head of a high-end boutique tour company. But taking on all that responsibility is exhausting. I never realized the psychological toll it took, until recently. I recognized that I needed to take care of myself because of my daughter's mental health requirements.

Now, as I've passed my 60th birthday, for the first time in my life I've been diagnosed with depression. And with suicidal ideation.

If that sounds like a downer, well, it can be, but I've taken it as a bull I need to grab by the horns and wrestle to the ground — and I'm not even in Spain (this week, at least). I've taken up my overachiever "problem" and turned it into a tool for good. I've thrown myself wholly into understanding mental illness, to helping others and raising awareness — and to saving myself.

So far so good. I'm still here and, aside from the dark moments, I'm approaching it all with my usual passion, compassion, and sense of humor. I recognize the comic potential in my own story. I'm, shall we say, risk averse. I'll often take food with me on exotic journeys — this is partly because you can't be sure to find a kosher meal in, say, Mongolia, but also because I like to play it safe. I prefer known quantity international hotel brands. I find food markets sort of icky: I've seen one too many exotic, and theoretically edible, penises (tiger, shark ... possibly also tiger shark) hanging there for sale. I'm a big fan of frozen yogurt. It's a low-risk treat.

My risk management and overachiever tendencies are in full view when it comes to my decision to save myself. One therapist isn't good enough. At one point I saw ten, seeing different therapists for different things. When I decide I'm going to take care of myself, I *really* take care of myself. I'm always all in. My absolute, in-built refusal to fail has helped keep me alive. Suicide would amount to failure. And I couldn't *live* with that.

This book you're now holding combines a global travelogue with the search for mental wellness, which is ultimately a search within yourself. I'm a veteran traveler, travel counselor, and advisor for a high-end, boutique company that specializes in travels for Jews and to places of Jewish interest. I also ran the North American wing of one of Israel's premiere private airlines for many years. Books on mental health and the search for happiness and wellbeing — a hugely popular category — have rarely crossed over with the likewise popular travelogue genre. This book inhabits that sweet spot on the Venn diagram, while also tapping into an interest in Jewish identity.

Only later in life, approaching sixty, did I receive a diagnosis of depression. This suddenly reshaped how I viewed my life as I'd lived it, the ups and downs. But it also came at a time when my daughter began suffering from mental health issues, and I started to have suicidal ideation. Rather than retreat, I stormed forward to learn all I could about my condition, to spread awareness of mental health issues to a broader public. This combined with my lifelong project of seeing the world: not in a sprint of project, but as the marathon project of a lifetime. During my travels I observed what made people happy in different countries and learned most of all about myself, looking outward, traveling the planet to wind my way to the journey within.

The result is this book. It comes from the heart. It's (hopefully) humorous. It's the story of traveling the world to find peace with one's own mind. It may be my story, but it's also universal — it can apply to any of us who have run across the rocks of mental wellbeing. I hope it brings comfort and perhaps a touch of inspiration. It's a happy story about a sad subject.

It's also packed with useful bonus material, like tips from a seasoned traveler and travel agent: when to book, which seats to ask for, what to look for in hotel inspections, how best to travel post-Covid, how to intentionally get bumped and earn money doing so, eating well on planes. But the core and heart of this book might best be described with the following equation.

World Travel + A Mental Health Journey + Judaism + Helping Others = Stuart Katz

Good news! You've been bumped up to first class on this worldwide tour. Drinks service will commence shortly. And don't forget to fasten those seatbelts.

Chapter 2

Almost Dying Will Do That to You

Make not your thoughts your prisons.

— **William Shakespeare**

The saying goes that just because you're paranoid, doesn't mean they're not out to get you. I feel that applies to me, but with a twist. My neurosis of choice isn't paranoia. What exactly it is may be best for you to decide, but suffice to say that I have a healthy respect for my own health and that of my loved ones, and I'm all too aware of the fragility of both body and mind. We'll get to the whole "fragility of mind" part. That's what most of this book is about. But we're just warming up, right? So how about we get started with an appetizer of fragility of body?

Blood clots are the bane of frequent, long-distance flyers. Sit too long and a clot can form in one of your legs, break off, then float on up and attack various internal parts. The lungs, for instance, which results in a pulmonary embolism. Yeah, I had one of those. Actually three, if we're being precise: a triple pulmonary embolism.

I fly a lot. That's the understatement of the century. I'm in the air for more than a month a year. I'd just arrived in New York. I was forty-eight at the time, soon to be celebrating twenty-five years of marriage to Carol, and was picked up at the airport by one of my four children, Ilan. He was in New York just that one day, before heading off to work at a camp for children with special needs. My other son, Gilad, was also in New York that summer, volunteering for US Customs and Border Patrol. One of my daughters, Adina, was just heading off to Canada to work at Camp Moshava, a Jewish summer camp, while my youngest daughter, Dafna, was taking a well-deserved break between a rigorous academic school year and her summer adventures. The whole Katz family is into travel, proactivity, healthy lifestyles, and being active in the expression and support of our Jewish faith. So, I was feeling proud and fulfilled and not the least bit under the weather when a renegade blood clot decided to hop on the highway from the leg up to my lungs.

Part of the problem was that I was so confident in my health, so un-paranoid about it, that I was oblivious to any symptoms that indicated that something problematic was afoot. If my son Ilan hadn't quite literally forced me to go to the ER, I would've shrugged it off and be dead now.

While I'm neurotic about many things in life (for instance, I hate driving over bridges), physical health isn't one of them. A case in point: I was at a Bat Mitzvah party. I usually can cut the rug and trip the light fantastic with the best of them, but my usual red hot dance moves were limited that evening. I remember wondering if I was getting old, but surely forty-eight isn't so old that you can't rock out to the most vibrant Hora ever performed or limbo with the best of them? The following week, I had periodic pain and difficulty breathing. Again, I didn't think much of it. Summer has always been the busiest time of year for my work, and it was fast approaching. I flew to New York with Dafna on a Monday in June 2011, and managed to work despite the continual, and it must be said increasing, pain.

By the time Saturday rolled around, I was feeling even worse, but I chalked this up to exhaustion. I had missed my traditional Saturday afternoon Shabbat nap, which I've maintained as a happy tradition that also offset my hyperactive work ethic, which means getting only some four or five hours of sleep per night. Come Sunday morning, I was feeling queasy and weak, but I hit the gym anyway for my normal daily workout. I could only handle a third of the reps I usually do. Then I was seeing my tour groups off at the airport, feeling drained and out of it. I had to sit often to rest, something I'd never done in the past.

In retrospect, I can see that I could qualify for a Ph.D. in denial. Where was my glorious neurosis when I actually needed it?

That evening I went out to dinner with my father-in-law, Ilan, and Dafna. An hour into the meal the pain became unbearable and, frankly, unignorable. I'd never felt anything like it before. It wasn't the intensity so much as its unique contours — it was clearly something that was new to my body, which is never a good sign. But let it be said that I may be, occasionally, a little stubborn. Ilan insisted on taking me to the hospital, but I had other ideas. I was booked to "roast" a friend that night, in an event dubbed the Second Annual Stuart Katz Memorial Roast — that name was meant as a joke, but perhaps *nomen est omen* as they say? Thankfully, Ilan called in the reinforcements — my wife, Carol — and they convinced me to head to the hospital.

When I arrived, the attending ER physician told me, "Literally within hours of death." I'd put off the loud and clear warning signs for a week and had put myself in far greater danger. The Roast would have to wait.

I had a triple pulmonary embolism — a blood clot had formed deep within my leg (called deep vein thrombosis), broken off, and drifted northward to my lung. Such wayward clots can be harmless, or they can meander their way where they are most unwelcome, like the brain and the lungs, and lead to death with little to no warning. In my case, I had a series of clots move up to my lung, causing a sudden blockage of an artery within it.

I'm a natural-born organizer. That helps when you run a travel business. Also, when choosing hospitals to reluctantly investigate strange pains, it turns out. While Ilan shuttled me away to a hospital, I checked my GPS and suggested South Nassau Community Hospital in Oceanside, New York. As I arrived, I found myself worrying about my health insurance. I have Israeli insurance. Could that mean that this pain of mine was about to form an embolism in my life savings? At this point, I realized I was in trouble and dispensed with the cost-benefit analysis.

In I went, taken through many tests, blood and urine samples, scans, and such. Being competitive, I was secretly hoping to get an "A." I had this fantasy of the doctors coming in to say, "It's nothing, Mr. Katz. Why, a fine man like you is a picture of health. You'll live till 120 and should even consider joining the pro tennis circuit. Nurse, get a load of this urinalysis! I've never seen results so perfect!" Turns out the fantasy rolling through my head didn't match the results. A CT scan found three blood clots on the edge of my lung.

At 2:30 am on June 27, 2011, I was admitted to the hospital. I can tell you the last time I was a patient in a hospital. Exactly forty-eight years and one week earlier. That's right — this was the first time I'd been a patient since my *birth*.

I turned out okay. But my good health and fitness were revealed to be double-edged swords. The doctors said that being fit helped me survive. But it had also lulled me into a false sense of security. I was healthy, working out six or seven days a week — I was a warhorse who never got sick! I always opted for stairs over the elevator to get more steps in. I somewhat obsessively count steps each day, trying to best my own records. I never smoked, used drugs, or drank anything stronger than Diet Coke. I was a minimalist when it came to meds of any sort. I thought I knew what I was doing from a theoretical standpoint, too. I earned MPH and MBA degrees with a focus on Health Administration, for crying out loud. Add that to next year's Roast notes!

My lifestyle surely fended off many health problems, but blood clots are sneaky. They tend to form when you are seated for extended periods of time. This is why many health professionals recommend taking aspirin before a long trip. Aspirin has a side effect of thinning the blood, and this is sometimes enough to ward off unwanted clotting. Clots are sometimes referred to as "economy class syndrome," with cramped seating and the inability to shift one's position contributing to clot formation. I spend hundreds of hours per year on overseas flights. I have so many frequent flier miles that I upgrade to business class probably 80% of the time, for health now as much as comfort, but that's still a lot of sedentary flying. Prolonged immobility is the leading cause of deep vein thrombosis, which can lead to embolisms.

I was given medicine to thin my blood and dissolve the clots. I have this thing about not wanting to take any medicine that I don't absolutely have to, particularly pain killers. I feel wary of them, perhaps the addictive side is what really concerns me, but the pain got so bad that, on two occasions, I accepted painkillers. Otherwise, my stubbornness muscled me through. I was in the hospital for eight days and thankfully required no other treatment. I was used to eighteen-hour workdays, so I was trying to get things done from the hospital bed. The iffy Wi-Fi at South Nassau Community Hospital is likely intentional — it forced me to convalesce.

Six weeks after my hospital stay, I still wasn't fully recovered. I continued to have minor breathing difficulty and pains in my leg which began when I sat for more than fifteen minutes after an activity, like working out at the gym. I needed to remain on meds for at least six months. I was also told some sobering statistics. More than half of those who suffer one pulmonary embolism will experience them in the future. My deep veins are routed to my lungs and so clots can travel the same path again.

In terms of mitigating the risk of it happening again, the key is avoiding prolonged periods of immobility. If your job involves sitting a lot, get up and walk around and stretch every hour. Flex your feet and legs by pointing your toes up towards your head. Feel your calves stretch. Repeat frequently. When traveling, take hourly breaks and move around. This could be pulling over at a rest area on the highway or walking the aisles on an airplane. Consider wearing compression stockings when traveling or, if your doctor agrees, taking a baby aspirin on your travel day. Drink a lot of fluids when traveling but avoid alcohol and caffeine. Wear loose-fitting clothing.

All that sounds good, but that treats the woes of the body. What's the equivalent of wearing compression stockings and avoiding caffeine when it comes to one's mental health? Let's head back in time now to where those problems all began. Your travel guide — yours truly — is a citizen of the world in a far more literal sense than most. How often do you meet a Panamanian, Israeli, American triple citizen?

Chapter 3

A True International: My Life as a Panamanian American Israeli Jewish Citizen of the World

Panama

If you can't fly, run. If you can't run, walk. If you can't walk, crawl, but by all means, keep moving.

— Martin Luther King Jr.

You may have noticed that I strive to overachieve. Why have one passport when you could have three? Good enough just isn't good enough for me. I also tend to expect more from myself than I do from others. I'm happy to suggest things to others that I'd find difficult to implement on myself. Life and the mind are confusing bundles of contradiction.

I'll give you an example. I served five terms as president of two of the synagogues of which I've been a member. That might not sound like much, but you don't know the Byzantine machinations of the synagogue soap opera. When it came to treating myself, one therapist wasn't good enough, so I saw ten. When I decide I'm going to take care of myself, I go all in. I'm always all in, which has sometimes been a problem.

What I see myself as not doing, as failing to accomplish, appears to others as if I'm completing superhuman feats of activity. But inadequacy is in the eye of the beholder, and I'm ruthless with myself. This leads to tremendous feelings of guilt when I'm not doing what I feel should be done. And guilt can paralyze. I don't accept guilt from others — you couldn't make me feel guilty if you tried — but I serve myself up large helpings of it all too often. This has always been my biggest crutch. It has also been a motivator. The desire to *not* feel guilty propels, just as feeling too guilty can box you in.

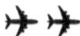

I was born in Panama to a Jewish family. My father was Panamanian, my mother American. My father's parents had escaped Europe. My grandmother was from Transylvania, Romania and my grandfather was from Hungary. They left Europe in the 1930s, sensing the impending cataclysm that would befall European Jews. Those family members who didn't leave were eventually murdered in the Holocaust.

They first emigrated to Cuba, then to Panama. My mother's parents were from Chicago. There was no Jewish school in Panama, so my father was sent to a Yeshiva, a Jewish boarding school, in Chicago. He met my mom then and they married very young. My father was twenty-one, my mother just nineteen. He enlisted in the US Army and requested to be stationed in Panama. So they moved to Panama when they got married. My brother and I were born there.

I grew up in the United States, but my first few years were spent in Colon, Panama. As a holder of three passports (having added Israeli citizenship), I'm a citizen of the world in the true sense. But my identity throughout has been more with my Judaism, the religion but also the culture, than with any particular nation.

So much of one's identity is linked to the dynamic with core family members at the earliest age, and yet we often don't realize it — including the potential long-term damage less-than-ideal dynamics that can be dished out — until decades later in life.

I was the oldest child (I've got a younger brother and two sisters), and the oldest grandchild, on both sides of my family. I use the word "child" hesitantly. I was, technically, a child, of course — who wasn't? But I didn't have a proper childhood because I was treated as an adult from infancy. At least, that's what my therapist says (yeah, one of those ten).

I feel as though my mother considered it an achievement that she produced four children in four years. Having checked that box, at a subconscious level it seemed like she "retired" from any further proceedings. She birthed us well enough, but then, despite her best efforts, seemed to have gone light on the nurturing-mommy-emotional-love part of the deal. Experts emphasize the importance of warmth, affection, and bonding between parents and their children. These early bonds lay the groundwork for healthy social, emotional, and cognitive development. This is why it is so important to educate ourselves and our children about taking care of the mental well-being of family members from a young age.

My parents provided all the material things we needed but didn't provide affection and emotional security. I only realized this much later. As in, many decades later. I guess deep down I felt that they loved me. But my understanding of love today is different from my understanding of it then. At the time, I didn't realize what was missing. I thought that my childhood was how all kids lived. Only recently, well into my fifties, did I start talking about our upbringing with my siblings. I'm sure that my parents believed that they provided us with an idyllic childhood. Sometimes we're so afraid of feeling guilty that we repel any attempt at apologizing or making amends. We'd rather dig in, not hear what our family has to say, than admit we could have done better — that's painful enough — and then feel guilty about it afterward — a far more lingering, tortuous affair. But that implies a consciousness on everyone's part, and that shouldn't be assumed.

One of the ways in which this manifests itself is in my hatred of birthdays. My birthday, anyway.

I've always hated my birthday. It's awkward because everyone knows I hate them, and they want to do something for me, but don't know what. I feel bad for my family and friends, as they're stuck. Every year, to this day, my parents send me a card specifically identifying just how old I've become.

I don't even remember birthdays as a kid. I assume it was celebrated in some way that I disliked so much that I've blocked it out. The first birthday I remember is my eighteenth.

I always felt that there were very high expectations of me, as early as age seven. From the perspective of most people, I could do no wrong. There was a presumptuousness on my parents' part that made me want to do wrong. But even when I didn't do well, they would find a way to say that I had, but without me feeling the emotional love.

It's hard to describe. I remember resenting that from the start. I wanted to see justice done. If I did poorly in school, I wanted it to be clear that I'd done poorly. I had a hard time accepting that my parents would only see what I did as a success. I was a seven-year-old grumpy adult.

The most egregious no-no that my parents practiced was corporal punishment. It's hard for me to fault them because they did what was, at the time, viewed as acceptable, though it's certainly not by today's standards. They were either showing off to their friends by praising my every move — whether I deserved it or not — or they'd hit me in punishment — whether it was warranted or not. It was a different era when such things were tolerated in a way that they would never be today, but that doesn't make it okay. I was hit a lot as punishment. Occasionally I understood why, that I'd done something wrong, but most of the time I felt that I was being hit for no reason at all.

As an adult, when my kids were already of college age, we had a traumatic family reunion. For the first time, I'd told my kids that my father hit us when my siblings and I were young. He would hit us, and my mother would be a spectator. He'd hit us, and she'd adjudicate, telling him that we'd had enough or that he should hit us more. My kids were shocked — two of them were studying psychology at the time, so they understood the effects of what I'd gone through better than I did. I was shaking. Then my mother brought out the potato kugel. Happy Hanukkah, everyone!

I was very close to all of my grandparents and adored them all, spending as much time as I could with them. I called both grandfathers Zaddie, which is "grandfather" in Yiddish. My father's father was Zaddie Katz, my mother's Zaddie Andelman. I called my grandmothers Bubbie: Bubbie Katz and Bubbie Andelman.

In Panama, we had a housekeeper who moved with us when we immigrated to the US. I cared about her very much and could tell how much she cared about me and my siblings. Recently, while writing this book, I took a trip to Panama and thought to see if I could get in touch with her, or at least her relatives (as I was quite sure she'd passed away by now). I wasn't successful, but it felt good to put in the effort to attempt to reconnect with someone who had been so important to my formative years. No matter how much time passes, the space in our hearts occupied by those who have been special to us remains.

She was our primary (almost exclusive) caretaker. She would remain with us until I was thirteen. The whole family would never eat together, aside from the Sabbath on Friday nights. The housekeeper would feed us kids separately from the parents. My parents loved entertaining, and we'd be assigned what to wear to dress up (often in matching sailor suits and saddle shoes — ick) and parade before the guests. But that was the only time we were allowed in my mother's all-white living room. My kids joke that this is why she loves Apple stores, with their all-white interiors. When the "parade" was over, we'd be shooed off to another room.

Travel was on my mind from an early age, as I used to enjoy plane-spotting (yup, just like trainspotting but you see if you can recognize plane models as they zoom past overhead) and I collected airline travel schedules for fun. My future occupation, running an airline, was surely in my blood.

We moved to San Diego, California when I was 4. When it was time for high school, aged thirteen, I was told I was going to a boys' boarding school, the same one that my father had attended. They found this very cool. Fulfilling my role as a legacy would check off another box on my parents' to-do list. There was no Jewish school within commuting distance of our house, and a Jewish education was of paramount importance to my parents — at all costs.

It was unhealthy for me to have been away from my parents at that early age. I was just too young. There was much crying for the first few weeks. It was the pre-cellphone age, of course. I'd call my parents from a public phone once a week, they came to visit me at school once a year, and I came home only twice a year. While I didn't feel great with my parents at home, I also hated boarding school. I felt like a layer cake of abandonment, parents with whom I didn't feel so good and then they packed me off to a school where I didn't feel so good.

The first year was awful, but then I adapted, and grew into the reality of being away from home, as I imagine many young students living far from their parents do. In retrospect it was probably good for me, maybe even did me a favor by providing that distance from my parents, space to grow. It gave me, or perhaps forced upon me, my independence at a very young age. But for the first year, I just hated it. I wanted to get out.

I remember standing in line for the payphone, crying. But I don't know if I actually wanted to go home, though I told my parents I did. When I was at home, I hated it there, too. Adding insult to injury, once I returned home on holiday to find that my parents had fired the housekeeper who had been with us since I was born — the person in the household to whom I felt closest. On the one hand, my parents were right: they let her go because we kids were older now and didn't need a caretaker. On the other hand, she felt more like a mother to me than my own mother did.

I pulled away from my parents as early as I could. They loved to brag about me, so I stopped telling them anything I'd done, as I didn't want to give them fuel to brandish my achievements as medals on their lapels. I don't think they ever did anything maliciously. They genuinely believed that their parenting was for the good. They also were very critical about my weight, as I was a chunky child (and later they were also critical of my children's weight). This was the probable cause of the unhealthy eating habits I've carried into adulthood. I've come to realize only late in life what a lot of baggage my siblings and I have lugged through the decades, weights borne because of what my parents did and didn't do. Even if the damage wasn't intentional, it's irreversible.

Is that legacy of weighty luggage what my father left me? I know that he loved me as my mother does as well, but I never *felt* it because I didn't feel it the way they intended for it to be felt. They had a skewed definition of what love is, what it means, which was not in sync with my own view.

I was in Los Angeles when I learned of my father's death, so I boarded a sixteen-hour flight to Modi'in, Israel. What stands out is my lack of feeling. I suppose I didn't care that he'd died, and that shot me through with guilt for that lack of feeling. Even in death, he could make me feel guilty for not caring that he was gone. Jewish guilt is a cliché, but there's truth to it. Like that saying about being paranoid. So too we could say that just because Jewish guilt is a cliché doesn't mean that we Jews don't have a special relationship with guilt. Catholics are famously wracked with guilt, too, but it's usually to do with concern that G-d or Jesus are going to find out that they've been up to no good. Jewish guilt isn't about G-d but about our interpersonal relationships. It's a terrestrial, secular self-flagellant.

I arrived at the cemetery. My mother and sister were there. His body was laid out, covered only with a sheet.

When I first saw his body, my gut reaction, the thing I thought of immediately, was that he could never hit me again. He hadn't hit me in more than four decades, but parental violence against children is an invisible scar that never heals. It smashes anything good they may have done for their kids.

At his funeral, the only people to speak were me and the rabbi. I opened with a quote from Mitch Albom's *Tuesdays with Morrie*: "Death ends a life, not a relationship." I managed to accentuate the positive in the eulogy and concealed the element of relief I felt at his passing, glossing over with the simple phrase "while there were challenging times …." Here is my eulogy:

> As I faced the past few weeks, the inevitability of not knowing when my father will pass, I knew that because of him and my grandparents, who I tremendously admired and loved and who laid the path for him, I will be able to get through it. All that I am, as a son, brother, husband, father, grandfather, and person, is not something that will end because of his death. More importantly, because I am my father's son and because of the relationship I had with him, I will carry it on in who I am and what I do in passing life's coping mechanisms to my children and grandchildren.
>
> My father leaves behind four children and fourteen grandchildren … Each of us will remember him in our own way. Each of us had a unique relationship with Dad … And who knows, maybe my Dad had favorites among his children or grandchildren, but my father treated us all equally and did his best to care for our physical needs all the same. He was passionate about nutrition and the many restaurant meals we shared always included a mini lecture on healthy choices at the restaurant. And often we would receive in the mail nutritional supplements that he thought we needed, and magazine articles that he thought were relevant to our health.
>
> Even more than the family, what he leaves behind is a legacy in the communities in which he was beloved, from Panama to

TRAVEL THERAPY

Chicago to San Diego to Modi'in. He could always be counted on to make the minyan (a term meaning "the quorum of ten men required for a prayer service and is sometimes used to refer to the prayer service itself"), read the Torah, daven for the Amud (a term meaning "to pray or lead services"), set up tables and chairs or whatever else was needed.

While there were challenging times, we each have some strong memories of him and perhaps we will think of those now.

Let me share some of the positive impacts he has had on me and that I find myself embodying in my everyday life. From him and my mom, I learned the importance of community work. From him, I learned the importance of hard work. From him, I learned the importance of providing for one's family. From him, I learned the importance of physical exercise and taking care of your body. From watching him, I learned how I could be a better father for my own children and what was needed to do so.

He had a determination and will which, at times, made him a force to be reckoned with. I have a strong work ethic and that is my tribute to him. From him, I learned that road rage isn't the norm — patience and acceptance is.

In the end, I am my father's son. What I take from that is not the emptiness felt at times. What I take from all that I experienced growing up, and what ultimately has shaped who I am, is what I learned from my dad. From an early age I worked, not because I wanted to but because my dad encouraged me to. From delivering newspapers to shoveling snow to scooping ice cream. The lesson I learned from this was simple: Work hard! Failure was never an option.

Picture a man strong and able and never asking for help. Now, picture a man slow to walk, having difficulties communicating, needing help. In all that my dad endured in the last six months of his life, I am learning that you can overcome adversity no matter the challenge. It is easy to quit when life has thrown challenges your way. You look at them and ask: Can I do this? Can I overcome this? From all that I have seen my dad go through, and no less important, all I have been going through, the answer is yes!

I have tried to pass on to my children and now grandchildren his best life skills: self-care, seeing the world, learning from others — not just in words, but in practice. I have learned through watching my father how to be more accepting of all people — regardless of race, age, or religion.

Given all this, I know that there are many things my dad accomplished and did throughout his life that I will never be able to do.

His last words to me, when we spoke on Sunday evening, were, "Everything is going to be okay — I don't know what Mommy is making a big deal about." Frankly, we never understood what Mommy was making a big deal about.

When I say, "I love you," to my children, which I try to do often, although certainly not often enough, I do so while remembering who showed me what those words could mean.

My father is now at peace. He's being reunited with my grandparents, from whom I learned so much. My hope is that, in some way, each person leaves here today honoring the best parts of themselves. These parts stem from our child parts and are protected by our adult parts. May this be the legacy that we can remember my father by. Let that be our tribute to him.

It was a eulogy that sought the best parts of the man, and there were good parts. The trouble is that we tend to internalize, to truly *feel* the not so good parts. They endure. The way kids think of parents is usually the way audiences at sporting events think about the referees. If they're doing everything well, nobody notices them or talks about them. The moment they mess up, they drill into our conscience, and we can't stand them. Parenting is the world's toughest job.

Neither I nor my three siblings were ever emotionally close to our parents. Growing up, we weren't best friends with each other, either. Today we're actually a lot closer. Not as a cohort, but one on one, we'd do anything for one another. It's an odd way to think about it, but that's how it is.

I still feel very much Panamanian. My kids love the Panama connection. When they fill out those slightly obnoxious sections of applications where they ask for your ethnicity, my kids love to put down "Hispanic."

Chapter 4

My Partner in the Journey of Life

Vancouver

The best and most beautiful things in the world cannot be seen or even touched — they must be felt with the heart.

— Helen Keller

Like so many "Hispanics," we'd lived in San Diego since I was four, so I chose to study at UCSD, University of California-San Diego. You might think that I would want to be anywhere else in the country other than where my parents lived. As there had always been to this point, there was a complicated dynamic. For financial reasons, the UC system made sense — California residents pay a very reasonable tuition, whereas private or out-of-state university is notoriously expensive in the US. My parents argued that they didn't want to pay for a dorm, and if I went to UCSD, then I could live at home. Just what I wanted to do! I was hoping for UCLA. Living in Los Angeles would have provided a cushion of distance that would've been good for me. But it was a matter of costs, and my parents were paying.

By this time, I was mature enough to set some boundaries. I spoke to my parents about how, if I were going to live at home, they weren't going to tell me what to do. I was eighteen at this point, but an 18-year-old who had lived away who was now moving back under his parents' roof is a different story. While I'd been at Yeshiva, my mother had taken over my bedroom and converted it into her office. I reclaimed it, but she was so in the habit of popping into the room whenever she felt like it, that she would appear unannounced, certainly without knocking, as if she'd forgotten that it was no longer her office. This was at a time when my siblings were all at boarding school themselves, so I was the only child at home, dealing with the parents full-on.

I spent as little time at home as possible. I started a branch of the national Jewish Zionist youth movement, Bnei Akiva, in San Diego. Between that and my classes and homework and the library (and beach time), I threw myself into working so I wouldn't have to be at home.

This was just at the start of airline frequent flyer programs, something I've loved and taken advantage of throughout my life. I saw it as a game, and I would try to beat the system. That all began while I was still a student. One of the tricks was booking a flight that you had a feeling would be overbooked, then arriving and allowing yourself to be bumped in exchange for a refund and frequent flyer miles. The best destination to reach from San Diego was Hawaii. There was one time when I flew to Hawaii — one of my favorite destinations — and back, three days in a row. I flew there in the morning, spent the day at the beach, then took the red eye back to San Diego, then flew back the next day, to do the same thing on another island. It was travel for the sake of travel because I'd gathered up those frequent flyer miles and didn't really need to go anywhere, so why not? I felt I had conquered travel and figured out the system enough to get to use it for free.

I was young and, in retrospect, behaving in a silly way. But it was fun and helped me understand how travel works, and that travel was an activity that I knew deeply enough to lead into a profession. I was still experimenting. For instance, I never was a fan of alcohol. Not interested in it. But when I was on the flight to Hawaii during one of those trips, I was offered a Mai Tai. Mai Tais have very little alcohol in them, but it was too much for me. I wound up taking an aspirin and this wasn't a winning combo. I was barfing for hours. That was one of my first drinks of alcohol and I didn't take another sip until I was in my late thirties. I am a cheap date. Everything seems to affect me more powerfully than it does others. When I've had surgery, I tell the anesthesiologist to give me half the normal dose and I'll be out like a light.

My college years were great. UCSD was a highlight. I grew close to some of my professors. Some I'm still in touch with today. The only thing I didn't like was the humanities requirement in the first year. I'm not a humanities guy. But the problem was really the professor. He ruined humanities for me, turned it into a trauma trigger. On the first day of class, he walked into the lecture hall, and said, "There are 300 of you here wanting to get an A. One of you will get an A. Two will get a B. Maybe twenty-five of you will get Cs. The rest of you? I'll see you next Fall …." I wasn't excited about humanities before that statement, but the idea that a professor would kick off a class by sucking all the optimism out of the room and promising that most of us would fail and have to take the class over again was not good bedside manner.

That class did prompt in me a devil-may-care streak that I don't otherwise associate with my personality. I figured that I was certain to fail the class, so why try? The final paper asked us to write an essay proving the existence of G-d. That was forty years ago and I'm not sure university professors can get away with that today without inciting the students to riot. But back then I literally took twenty-five sheets of blank paper, stapled them together, and wrote my name on the first page. That was it. My submission. My biggest internal debate was: To staple or not to staple? That was the question. My instinct told me not to staple them, but I was afraid they'd get lost. I ended up with a B.

While at UCSD, I spent my extracurricular time working with Bnei Akiva. It grew quickly to over 300 members in two years, which is a lot for a movement of this type in a place without a big Jewish population. I was in touch with the movement's national coordinators and convinced them that I needed some help, thanks to the expansion of the numbers in our local chapter. They sent out a young couple from New York, three years older than I was, to spend a year in San Diego helping me. It went so well that, at the end of the year, I was appointed national director of the movement, based in New York. The couple offered plenty of advice on what to do in New York, whom to call, where to live. They also had a list of people who were members of the movement and mentioned this one girl who was into literature and would be a really good person to help introduce me to New York. I took notes and prepared to move across the country.

I finished UCSD and took advantage of heading to New York by doing a Masters in Public Health at Columbia University. In San Diego, I'd interned at Planned Parenthood. I'd often be asked why I was interested in helping in the field. I'd never known someone with an unwanted pregnancy, but I was fascinated with the topic, the Roe v Wade debate. Most people I knew were against legal abortion, while I was for a woman's choice, so I felt I was supporting an important cause and was part of the underdog team. I had gone from great experiences with UCSD professors (that humanities teacher aside), who really felt like mentors, to Columbia professors who felt like the opposite — they'd show up an hour late to a three-hour seminar as if they didn't value our time. Then they'd say, "You guys know what you have to do. I might be a little late next time." I didn't feel like I learned anything from the professors. I'd just paid for a piece of paper that says I have a degree from Columbia. That has a value for resumes, but it didn't feel good.

Meanwhile, my work for Bnei Akiva continued. I had to find a new editor for a children's newsletter the organization produced. It occurred to me that this girl who was into literature might be a good candidate. A friend of mine from Los Angeles who was also new to New York was dating her roommate. I met her — Carol — and offered her the editor gig. She said she was honored, and I replied, "Great, let's meet for dinner to talk about it." Turns out she asked my LA friend to find out what I'd thought of her. It was a positive review, but nothing more happened at that point.

A short time later, I was running a leadership weekend for the movement in Chicago, and Carol was part of it. Sparks sparked and we've been together ever since. I remember telling her, very clearly, that I planned to be traveling for the rest of my life. I said she was welcome to come along for the journey. She was up for it, but she'd hardly traveled at all. She'd been on a plane just once, to go to Israel. Otherwise, her travels to date had been by station wagon around the US, once across the country to California, once down the East Coast to Florida, staying at Motel Sixes. That was about it.

Carol's parents were cautious. I overheard her mom telling her not to go anywhere with me until she had got a ring on her finger. That didn't take long.

I took our relationship seriously from the start. We wound up getting engaged after about a year of dating. During that time, I wrote her eighteen poems and sent her roses on eighteen occasions — eighteen stands for "life" in Hebrew.

As national director of the movement, I was traveling a lot. I loved that aspect of it. This meant that I worked closely with a travel agency. The agency was planning a Halloween party in New York — or so I claimed. Now, as an Orthodox Jew, I'm not really supposed to do Halloween, but what the heck, right? Carol was up for going, we'd buy costumes, it'd be fun. I told her to meet me at the terminal at JFK airport. I knew she loved the Knight in Shining Armor concept, so that was the costume I chose. It was a big surprise, as she'd forgotten she'd told me this dream of hers.

She came as a witch. When she arrived, I'd set up a treasure hunt in the terminal. She followed one clue after another. It was great fun. The fourth clue led to the top of the old Pan-Am terminal. That was where I proposed to her.

We got married in September 1986 and went on a series of honeymoons. The first was to Vancouver to visit the World's Fair. At the fair, you could get these passports and have them stamped at various international exhibits there. I said, "We'll start here, but then we'll go around the world and get our real passports stamped for real."

The plan was to go camping in Vancouver, Carol was, at the time, much more outdoorsy than I (we've since grown used to domestic comforts, so our camping period was very brief). My idea of "camping" is staying at a Motel Six instead of a Hilton. I'd told her, "Look, because of the World's Fair there are no hotel rooms available in the city, so we're going to camp." Carol was suspicious that I wouldn't actually go camping with her, but she'd overheard me telling my grandfather that we would be camping. Carol told this to one of her friends and said, "He's not going to lie to his Zaddie." So she was sure I was up for it — my first time in a sleeping bag, and all that. In Vancouver, we got into a taxi, and I told the driver to take us to this campground. Only I knew that it was right across the street from a hotel and a marina. She still thought we were going to a campground.

We were dropped off and entered this little office. The guy inside says, "I'll take you to your cabin." So now she's thinking that we're staying in a log cabin or something. Then he takes us to a cabin — on a boat. I didn't think I'd be able to sleep if we actually went camping, so staying on a boat was the roughest I could handle.

After Vancouver, we set out for the former Soviet Union: Russia, Moldova, and Ukraine. You see, our honeymoon wasn't just about romance. We were actually on a secret mission.

Chapter 5

All My Honeymoons

Moscow

But they who wait for the Lord shall renew their strength; they shall mount up with wings like eagles; they shall run and not be weary; they shall walk and not faint.

— Isaiah 40:31

What a honeymoon! First *nearly* camping in Vancouver, then being interrogated by Soviet police in Odessa!

While Vancouver was just about fun, there was more to our next honeymoon stops than romance and discount kosher meals. We were off to Russia, Moldova, and Ukraine. I'd say we were the perfect cover for covert activities — we appeared totally inept. In fact, we were genuinely inept, but somehow managed to not get into (too much) trouble — and actually fulfilled our secret mission.

Our mission was to bring brochures, books, information, and messages to Jews isolated behind the Iron Curtain. It sounds grander than it was, but we were secret emissaries for the Zionist movement. The material we smuggled with us was all related to Judaism and Israel, with the goal to instill hope for the future within them. The idea that, one day, they would be able to live freely as Jews in the State of Israel. This was a subject that we were not allowed to speak about publicly until 2002, but now our actions can be discussed. At the time, only our parents knew what we were really up to.

The goal was to bring hope to Jews stuck in a regime and environment that ran from tolerant to dismissive to abusive when it came to the attitude toward Jews. Pre-internet, pre-messaging software, messages were sent through the post or hand-delivered. The postal system was monitored in the Soviet Union, so packages sent from Israel or the US were unlikely to reach their destinations and were likely to get the addressees into trouble. I suppose you could call the Zionist network an underground movement. We were chosen to be emissaries. We were interested in traveling to the Soviet Union anyway, so why not bring along some suitcases packed with illicit materials, while we were at it?

You shouldn't imagine us as a pair of James Bonds with microfiche hidden in our socks. What we brought was all rather innocuous: posters of Israel, song sheets in Hebrew, Judaic objects like menorahs (eight-stemmed candelabras used in the Hannukah tradition), kiddush cups (formal cups used in the traditional prayer over wine as part of Shabbat), Havdalah sets (used in a ritual to mark the end of Shabbat), tallitot (fringed prayer shawls), tefillin (leather boxes containing scrolls inscribed with prayers) and Israeli flags (a practice I continue to this day when I travel, giving them out to people the world over — more on that later). The idea was to provide materials that would keep the spark of Judaism alive and the hope that those who wished to do so could eventually emigrate to Israel. There was a general term for them: *refuseniks*, those who had been denied permission to emigrate. This encouragement to emigrate was seen as subversive activity by the KGB, who took an unwanted interest in us.

We didn't have any special training. The Zionists from the US who gave us the material only insisted that we memorize the names and addresses of the people in the Soviet Union to whom we were supposed to deliver the goods, to avoid the risk of carrying a list with us. We had no smartphones, of course, and it was too dangerous to write down the addresses, should our belongings be searched or confiscated. So the only real spy craft was to memorize a whole lot of names and addresses. To do so, we had to learn the Russian alphabet

"Cyrillic" and some (very) basic Russian. This felt like a fun challenge at the time — we were young and naïve enough not to be terrified. It's ironic that, at the time, I was more scared of driving across a bridge (with the expectation that any bridge I might happen to cross will suddenly collapse for no reason at all) or ordering unidentifiable and potentially overly spicy food than to infiltrate the Soviet Union as a secret agent. So it goes with neuroses: We tend to focus on and dread implausible dangers to the point where we can blissfully cruise past real ones.

We maintained our cover by visiting touristy things you're supposed to do when visiting a place like Russia. I'm not much for culture. I don't like opera. I hate ballet. No circuses for me, thank you. We had to attend a performance of *Anna Karenina*, which was one of my worst punishments — but we'd look suspicious if, as American tourists, we didn't attend a ballet, right? *Everyone* loves a ballet. Well, almost everyone. I have zero appreciation for the arts.

People would come up to us and we'd have to figure out if they were KGB agents or sympathetic souls. Carol wore a Star of David necklace, which was a beacon for refuseniks who we were supposed to meet, but also for KGB agents.

At the time, the US and Soviet Union were on slightly friendlier footing, thanks to the Reykjavik Summit, so it seemed like as low-key an opportunity as any. In October 1986, President Ronald Reagan and General Secretary of the Soviet Union, Mikhail Gorbachev, were meeting in Iceland to chat about banning all ballistic missiles, while Reagan was all for militarizing outer space. The deal was meant to be that the USSR would stop its missile program if the US would stop theirs and give up the dream of shooting at enemies from space. Gorbachev just wanted to talk about arms control, but Reagan threw in other elements, from human rights to the Soviet invasion of Afghanistan to — and this is where we came in — permitting Soviet Jews and dissidents to emigrate. It didn't go smoothly, but it was still more amicable than the superpowers had been in ages. So why not take the opportunity to smuggle goodies to those Soviet Jews who hoped to head off to Israel in the near future?

We did have a cover story of sorts if we were caught. We would say that we were strictly on a personal mission from our rabbi back in the US. We genuinely thought that we wouldn't be in any actual danger. At least, the goal was for us not to be in any danger. We imagined that the worst thing that could happen to us was that we'd be kicked out of the country and sent packing back home. Our "handlers" back in the US and Israel, if we can call them that, said that we wouldn't be sent to prison and that our lives would not be in danger. If we were arrested and accused of being spies, we should just tell them we have no idea what they're talking about. Who were we to disagree?

Carol and I were aware that we were being watched, noted by various Soviet police and some plainclothes, shifty agent-ish types. But they left us alone as we made our rounds, seeing sights, playing the role of newlywed tourists (which we were, of course), and making our covert deliveries. The first tough encounter came in Odessa, fourteen days into our trip.

We were supposed to visit a family, the husband of which had been arrested and sent to Siberia. We were trying to help the wife and husband get in touch. They'd been married for four weeks before he was taken away and it had been six months since they'd been in contact. We had memorized a photo of her and knew where she lived. We'd been briefed that it was a good modus operandi to identify our contacts while they were jogging in the park. We would jog alongside them briefly, long enough to exchange information and plan a later rendezvous, before separating. No one would be the wiser.

One day we spotted her out jogging in a park. I jogged alongside her to make initial contact. This is how we conversed without, I thought, being spotted. For three days we were jogging partners. We never went to her apartment because she thought it might be bugged and we thought the KGB were onto us. Finally, after three days, she said that she didn't care what happened to her and we were invited to her apartment. This must be counted as a success — we eventually ran into her when she moved to Israel, years later. So, I suppose, mission accomplished!

We were visiting a different person's apartment in Odessa when there came a knock at the door. It was the KGB.

Oopsy.

Our hearts dropped into our stomachs. They took me and Carol away in a paddy wagon.

A pair of police officers escorted us not to the police station, but into the hotel where we were staying. They led us into a ballroom in which some thirty police officers sat in a circle, smoking. They sat us down in the middle of the circle as the police puffed and puffed at their cigarettes. I'm not sure if this was a tactic to "smoke us out" or simply a confluence of enthusiastic smokers, but it made us feel sick, nearly choking on all the smoke. I'm sure it was tactical to have police seated all around us, making us feel vulnerable beneath their stares. We were at the center of the circle and couldn't see all the agents behind us — it was intentionally disorienting.

They spoke to us together in the ballroom, but then separated us, just like they do in the movies, hoping, I suppose, to catch us giving different versions of our story. We hadn't really rehearsed for this. We stuck to our predetermined story. They kept on asking why we were there, asking the same question in different ways, taking different approaches, hoping we'd accidentally let slip the truth or contradict ourselves. My mother used the same tactic when she wanted to know what I was up to. But we didn't slip up, as far as we know.

We probably should have been scared. Neither of us recalls being so. It was as if it were all happening in a movie, in someone else's life. The only thing that bothered us was the chain-smoking of the policemen. We hate the smell of cigarettes. And, true to cinematic form, the Soviet police were billowing wafts of cheap tobacco smoke in these closed rooms. I guess they had nothing solid or didn't feel up for making an international incident of it, so they let us go. We probably should have quit while we were ahead, but this gave us a boost of confidence in our latent secret-agent-ness.

After Odessa, we headed to Kharkov in Ukraine. That's where we met the KGB face-on for the second time. So much for the secret-agent-ness.

We knew nothing about Kharkov, and there was no Google Maps at the time to figure out how to get there, and where to go once we were there. We made our way to the city and wanted to buy a map, to orient ourselves, but we couldn't find a single one that covered all of Kharkov.

Here we were supposed to pose as university students, as Kharkov is a university town. But we'd already been in the region for nearly two weeks and, clearly, the KGB had caught on. There were maps of Kharkov, you see, but no one wanted to sell us any (I imagine James Bond had similar problems). We went to every newsstand and bookstore we could find. No maps. From the looks in the eyes of the vendors when we asked for maps, we understood that the jig was up. We were under surveillance.

We knew that we should call it quits, but we still had a few stops to make. It helped that the proverbial ice had been broken and we were aware that we were being followed. Our youthful naivety, and the fact that we'd gotten out of one police interrogation none the worse for wear, gave us more confidence, rather than scaring us into a quick exit.

They must have figured out where we were intending to go. We'd finally find an address in Kharkov, but the numbers on the buildings would be missing right where we thought we were supposed to be to meet with a refusenik. We'd be on a big avenue, and we'd see number ten and number twenty-two, but we're looking for number seventeen and all the house numbers around the one we're looking for had been removed from the buildings. We eventually found the house, but I was freaking out. It was like they could read our minds and were working a step ahead.

Our next stop was Kishinev, in today's Moldova. We employed the same modus operandi. But that's where the KGB picked us up. Again.

They took us to their station this time and asked us what we were doing here. Now old hands at being interrogated, we stuck to the script. The agents would talk together in Russian, and we had only a few words and phrases, but I decided to use them.

I said, "I want ice cream."

An agent replied, "No ice cream."

Then I said, "I really need ice cream."

And he's staring at me, wondering, what the heck is going on? I'm not supposed to speak Russian, I'm supposed to be scared, and I'm insisting on getting ice cream.

That was the only thing I could remember how to say.

Perhaps my ice cream tactic successfully sowed seeds of confusion (or convinced them that we were idiots incapable of doing anything subversive). After about four hours, they let us go. As they dropped us off outside the city train station, one of the agents wagged his finger at us and said, "No more." This seemed like a reasonable request, given the circumstances, but we were scheduled to go on to Chernovtsy (now Chernivtsi, in the border region between today's Romania and Ukraine). Looking back, I'm not sure if they just decided we were innocent or decided that whatever we were doing wasn't sufficiently sinister to warrant an international debacle. Or maybe they identified us as sufficiently inept not to be a threat.

Carol's birthday fell during our trip while we were in Moldova. It was her first birthday as my wife, so I wanted to get her something nice. But when it came to shopping in the former Soviet Union in the 1980s, it was more about what limited items happened to be available on a given day. Selection wasn't a luxury. If that was the day when a truckload of woolen mittens arrived, then that was what there was to buy. Moldova in 1986 wasn't exactly a shopper's paradise. So I was trying to figure out what to buy for Carol. I set off to the central market in the town we were visiting as part of our secret mission and got chatting with a local vendor. The pickings that day were slim.

"I can sell you a chicken," he helpfully offered.

"Is it kosher?"

"Well, it's not *not* kosher."

"What does that mean?"

"It's not dead yet."

I settled for a story as my gift. A story of almost buying Carol a live chicken for her birthday. Everyone loves a good story, right?

In Chernovtsy, I was out for a walk on my own, when I spotted my KGB "minder." He was following me conspicuously, and I had nowhere in particular to go at the time, so I decided to mess with him. I wound up walking back and forth along a single long block for over an hour. The KGB agent was getting more and more furious, but I kept on leading him in circles. I guess I thought it was fun and was giving him some passive-aggressive just desserts. Well, at a certain point, he had enough and decided to become active-aggressive. He knocked me to the ground and stormed off. I guess it served me right for treating something that was quite serious and could have potentially led to my long-term imprisonment, as a game. This physical encounter sobered me up on that front.

Fortunately, by that point, we could actually say, "Mission accomplished." We'd delivered the Zionist contraband to all the memorized addresses. When I felt the airplane's wheels rise off the tarmac, on our flight away, a knot I hadn't been aware of inside my stomach suddenly unwound. I'd been more nervous than I'd realized and was grateful to have made it out safely — a feeling I would have in the future numerous times, particularly when I would travel as a disaster relief volunteer. The wheels rising off the runway, then whirring into their enclosure in the belly of the plane. That's a sound I associate with comfort and thanks.

We flew to Copenhagen to refresh ourselves. The relief of being there remains a physical association I have with the city. Then we came back home.

The Jews we'd visited were always very grateful, especially the refuseniks who were more active in the Zionist community, most of which was underground in the USSR. They recognized the risk we took, maybe more than we had.

It would be nice to think that our efforts helped the cause. From 1981–1987, a reported total of 24,542 Jews emigrated from the Soviet Union, most of them headed to Israel. We were there in October 1986. But from 1988–1992, the total spiked up to 642,265 (the number blossoming from 1991, when the Soviet Union was dissolved). We did our part and that felt good. It also feels good, in retrospect, that we didn't end up in prison, where there would have been a great deal more unpleasant cigarette smoke to contend with. On the positive side, had we been imprisoned in the Soviet Union, I would've had an ideal opportunity to learn Russian!

Chapter 6

TAL Tours: How to Run a Travel Agency

38,000 Feet

The worst loneliness is to not be comfortable with yourself.

— Mark Twain

As a child who enjoyed plane-spotting and collecting airline travel schedules, maybe my future profession was written in the stars! I remember the stack of those printed airline schedules. The crisp bend of brochures, the firm paper stock they used, the glossy covers, the pill shaped and colored airplanes, the infinite possibility of world travel, the promise of a machine that permitted the superpower of flight. All that sounded pretty great to this seven-year-old. I also loved the playing card packs they gave out on flights, the little soaps I'd collect from each airline, even the baggage check tags. Not only did I collect airline schedules, but I would memorize them. This led to my interest in plane-spotting. I would hear the distant roar of an engine and rush outside, craning my neck to the sky, shielding my little eyes from the sun, and try to identify the plane that flew overhead. Was it a Boeing 747? A 707? A British Aerospace model? An Airbus A300? It was icing on the cake if I could identify not only the plane but, with my stack of schedules in mind, I'd check the kitchen clock and could also tell where the plane was going to or coming from.

Growing up, travel by plane was always a highlight, a special treat I looked forward to. I've always had the travel bug. The journey was as much fun as seeing new lands, meeting people from different places, glimpsing new cultures. I wanted to learn from others, learn how others did things differently. I feel that there's a level of tolerance, even acceptance, for differences in humanity that travel promotes. You realize that there are other ways to live than the one you're used to, and it helps you keep perspective and respect otherness. I'm a big believer that there's no enemy but ourselves. When, later in life, I would deal with my own mental illness, this slogan of mine switched from metaphorical to literal. But early on, I saw it as a practical idiom. Our own intolerance, the expectation that our way is the only "right" way, that others should shift to meet our expectations, is the problem. In short, *we* are our own problem. The issue isn't out there but within.

Even while thinking this, I spent my life traveling and looking for self-actualization, a feeling of doing good, a reason to exist, through external interactions. This was most obvious in my serial do-gooding as a humanitarian volunteer. I'll hear about a crisis — a tsunami, an earthquake, a hurricane, a tidal wave of refugees — and I'll feel the compulsion to help, in person. This is a good thing. But it's also a neurotic thing, the extent to which I do it.

This is a manifestation of what therapists call "work" or "productivity dysmorphia." Whatever I do is never enough in my own eyes. Objectively, if you ask someone else, they think I'm hyper-productive and do plenty. I'm the only one who is never satisfied with myself. "Dysmorphia" as a mental illness is most often associated with "body dysmorphia," an objectively incorrect belief that some aspect of one's body is the wrong size or shape. But it is a term applied to other aspects of life. It's like looking at the world through a funhouse mirror — your view is skewed but you cannot convince yourself otherwise, no matter what others tell you, no matter how much you are presented with objective evidence that all is well.

Even writing this book required multitasking. I'll be typing away but also checking email every few minutes and chatting on WhatsApp and even occasionally on-call for a suicide prevention hotline. I can't seem to do just one thing, because even if I do that one thing well, I feel like I'm not doing enough. So I've gotten good at juggling many things and doing all of them reasonably well. But it's exhausting. I know it is, but I can't help it.

This dysmorphia manifests in my work and feelings of productivity, but I have what might be called "philanthropic dysmorphia," which I would define as a feeling that no amount of volunteer work, no number of people helped, is ever enough. This is a good thing to be compulsive about — better that I can't stop helping people than, say, can't stop drinking alcohol. I recognize that I am lending a hand in a world where too few people proactively help others. But I always feel I've not done enough. Guilt is like some invisible, rabid rat trailing me, biting at me, and disappearing only while I'm in the midst of a bout of hyper-productivity, especially when volunteering to help others. The moment I stop, there he is again, chewing into me the idea that I should have done more.

I'd also throw myself headlong into volunteer situations that were potentially dangerous for me, particularly if those I wished to help weren't necessarily keen on being helped by a Jew. An example was the Syrian refugee crisis. I felt strongly that humans helping humans was always a good thing, but I'd have friends warn me that I might get myself killed trying to help. My attitude was: I don't care who you are, but if you're in trouble, I want to help you.

Volunteer work aside, my wanderlust is another symptom of the ultimate diagnosis — that I wasn't happy with myself. But it took decades, and a gaggle of therapists, for me to realize this. For the next few decades, I would be traveling and traveling and traveling some more. One of my "homes" was at around 38,000 feet. I've spent more time in airplanes than many have in homes they've lived in.

The idea of turning pro with my love for travel hadn't occurred to me. In middle school, I volunteered during the summers at a local travel agency, just to see what it was like. I worked there for modest pay during some later summers, and I really enjoyed it. Then I went to college and to grad school, and it never really occurred to me to make travel my profession. I'd helped organize some Jewish group trips that had gone well, and I enjoyed the feeling of having everything under control, sorting out problems, putting out fires — being the overachiever who could please and impress others. I'd plan trips for friends for fun. They'd tell me where they wanted to go, and I'd do the research to find the best deals. This was before websites like booking.com or kayak.com did it for you. Long before. The fax machine had just come out. I spent $2,500 on one of these "cutting-edge" devices. I was so proud of it, happy for any chance to put it to use.

I love a good deal. Whether or not I really need what I'm getting, I'm on a runner's high when I know I've found a great price. That is why I have an improbably large collection of Gonzaga sweatshirts. As a practicing Jew, I did not attend the Catholic Jesuit Gonzaga University. But they make very comfortable sweatshirts, and I found a sweet deal on them, so I keep acquiring Gonzaga merchandise. It's surprisingly good as a conversation starter, too. My paths seem to have crossed with an inordinately high percentage of Gonzaga alumni, as I'm often greeted, especially in airports, by folks reacting to my sweatshirts.

This quirk of mine also extends to an almost pathological love for bartering. The process is so much fun for me that I'll negotiate at market stalls for items I don't actually want to buy — then that guilt kicks in and I'll buy them anyway. In Singapore, I bought a whole wardrobe's worth of clothes that it turned out I really didn't need because I got a good deal. But when my luggage was lost on my way to a meeting in Milan, I couldn't bring myself to buy anything, because everything was full price.

Carol and I were living in Dallas and working for Bnei Akiva. We were young — I was twenty-five. I had a Master's in Public Health and an MBA, so I figured I'd get a job, but I didn't have any in mind.

Then I got a call from a travel company in Israel. At first, I thought, "Hey great." Because we were thinking of moving from Dallas to Israel and this seemed like the perfect opportunity. They would be in Dallas soon enough and wanted to meet me. When we met, they said, "We've heard all about you. We've seen what you've done. And we do trips to Israel. We want you as part of our team." Someone at Bnei Akiva had referred me, and I'd actually worked with them, but hadn't realized it. Their agency coordinated ground travel arrangements in Israel for Bnei Akiva groups. They'd just been given a contract to coordinate all aspects of the Bnei Akiva trips to Israel. This couldn't be any more perfect, could it?

Well, almost. They wanted to open a US branch in New York and asked if I'd be interested in running it.

I didn't want to move to New York (it's not for everyone and certainly not for me), but I did want to be involved. They offered a robust salary, but I just didn't want to go there. These were the days when you had to be in specific key locations to do work. Today, with the internet and mobile phones, the work world is a lot more flexible. Now, I might be able to run a travel agency in New York from a home in Israel. Back then you had to be boots on the ground where the action was, even if you were the proud owner of a $2,500 fax machine. So it was New York or nothing.

With a fixed idea that I wouldn't move to New York, I moved to New York. Such is life. Their improved offer was too good to pass up — I'd move there for two years and take on a 30% partnership stake in the company. That was significantly more attractive than a straight salary. I agreed — on condition that I could live in Israel after the first two years. And I would still keep my salary in US dollars, which was also very attractive, since the Israeli economy at the time was shaky. We had a kid and a half at the time (our firstborn, born in Dallas, plus a "bun in the oven," as they say). Essentially, it was an offer I couldn't refuse.

Now, I didn't know the first thing about running a travel agency. I'd organized group tours, but that was it. I knew how to sell airline tickets and create itineraries for clients. I really enjoyed it, was even passionate about it. But that's more the role of a travel agent, not the director of a travel agency, who has all manner of bureaucratic, managerial things to worry about.

New York is a polarizing city. Many love it: the constant action, the crowds, the lights, the traffic, the edginess, the grime. Many hate it because of the constant action, the crowds, the lights, the traffic, the edginess, the grime. I'm in the latter category. I had spent three years there while I was heading up the Bnei Akiva National Office and, at the same time, doing a Master's in Public Health at Columbia University. I was totally put off by it: too busy, too crowded, too pressurized. Definitely not where I'd want to raise a family. I'd get a bit sweaty at the thought of being a New Yorker. But it was too good a prospect to pass up, with no other strong options on the horizon.

So, New York it was. I established a company called TAL Tours and became its US national director. It was only going to be two years, after all.

Well, eighteen years later, we were still there. Best-laid plans, right? We were doing well financially, we were a family of six by that point and, as often happens, there's a degree of inertia, particularly if your lifestyle is comfortable.

After the first four years, the original partners who had hired me sold their shares of the company to a new, larger firm — a multinational based in

Israel, but with partners from Jordan and Egypt, as well. I didn't get along well with the new partners and didn't agree with their business approach. I remained for another four years, before deciding that I'd had enough.

My mantra has always been that I have to be happy with what I'm doing, or I'm going to stop doing it. Sounds logical enough, right? But you have to also consider what "happy" means.

I'm not a happy guy. I'm a content guy, most of the time, but I have periods of feeling down, and I'm often anxious. I think contentment is a reasonable life target. Happiness, in a euphoric, effervescent, bubbly, everything's-coming-up-roses, I can't wait for tomorrow but please never let today end because it's all so wonderful sense, is rare and childlike. Grownups, married for decades, with kids and mortgages, will find happiness a rare luxury, like spotting a Bird of Paradise after months trekking the jungle. Contentment, on the other hand, is dignified satisfaction with what you have, with your lot in life. It's a more Buddhist lack of desire, with a dash of Capitalism that says that I earn enough to afford that which I desire. It's a lack of need, your basics fulfilled, things going more or less according to plan, no raging turmoil (with the periodic and expected choppy waters of wedlock and parenthood considered acceptable). Working towards contentment is a reasonable and more achievable goal than striving for happiness.

America is a wonderful place, but its culture is laced with the promise of boundless happiness, too often equated with boundless financial riches (I consider this idea in greater depth in Chapter 15, on Bhutan, where they measure Gross National Happiness). It's an acquisitive culture: if you're not happy, the subconscious message goes, then it's because you need to buy more things or earn more money with which to buy more things or both. In my travels, I've seen how exceptionally rare American-style happiness is. Contentment is a goal out of reach for most of the world. Happiness doesn't even peak up over the horizon — this is a subject we'll discuss further near the end of the book. My volunteer work for humanitarian crises and refugee centers has shown me that sadness is far more natural to the human condition, alas, than happiness or even contentment. Humans struggle.

I'm one of the lucky ones. I have no financial worries. Or rather, I'm *always* worried about finances, but that's just me — I'm lucky to be financially stable by any international measure. I can live where I choose to. I'm free. I've got a loving family. I am content. And grateful.

But I've also got a darkness that sometimes melts over me. Now at the cusp of sixty, as I write these lines, I've learned that this was depression. I always thought that it was just a part of me, a part of life, a part of just about everyone. I am more anxious than I'd like to be, more than most people I know. But when I do volunteer work, not only do I feel good about helping others, but my own life is put into perspective.

Chapter 7

The $100,000 Fuel Bill: How to Run an Airline

New York

The best years of your life are the ones in which you decide your problems are your own. You do not blame them on your mother, the ecology, or the president. You realize that you control your destiny.

— Albert Ellis

There was an early experience of this melting darkness when I was in New York, no longer feeling comfortable working for the larger multinational that had acquired TAL Tours. Their modus operandi felt disingenuous, making me feel uncomfortable in my dynamic with clients, who I had to deal with face to face. You develop working friendships over the years. Clients need to trust you, or they'll go elsewhere. Travel doesn't involve monopolies — you must demonstrate your reliability to compete and, most of all, to retain clients.

On too many occasions, the company would promise the client one thing, then fail to deliver. That meant that I, often in person, was making promises to people I knew and often liked. Then, for reasons out of my control, my company would fail to deliver. They functioned in a way that I felt was unethical.

The breaking point came when they told me that they wanted to merge with another company in the US. The other partners entered my office, sat down, and said, "This is what we're going to do." Though I was a minority owner, it was presented as a decision I wasn't part of. I was being told. I replied, "That may be what you're going to do, but I'm not going to be a part of it."

That took them aback. I recognized that I was their primary asset. They did, too. Seeing that I was not going to be swayed, they came back and said, "Okay, then you can buy us out."

I was thirty-three at the time. I remember thinking, "I don't have the money to buy them out." But we talked it through and came up with an agreement that was feasible. We spaced out my payments over an extended period. I paid more than I wanted to, but less than they'd hoped for. I borrowed money and took on 100% ownership of the company.

It was my ship to run now.

The now ex-partners had wanted to go big. I felt it was best to remain small, specialized, and nimble. This helped me during the pandemic and ensured that I was able to personally oversee quality control and make sure that whatever TAL Tours promised clients, the clients would receive. Even today we're a small operation, with a handful of staff members, but when you work with TAL Tours, you'll be working with me, hands-on. We can quickly adapt to whatever the world throws at us, without the need for board meetings and the lumbering machinations of large companies.

TAL Tours has remained ever since and is still going strong. But there was also a period during my New York life when I took on an additional challenge.

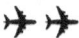

One of the original partners from our tour company, someone I remained close to, was tapped to be involved in a new Israeli airline. In 2003, shortly after I took over TAL Tours, he reached out to me and asked if I would open a US office, based in New York, for the airline, Israir, which is still in operation.

This old colleague came over to my office — we ran TAL Tours out of just two rooms on Long Island. He laid out the airline's plan. He deeply trusted me, and I felt good about working with him. It was certainly tempting. I love logistics and travel and the logistics of travel. This was a monster of a challenge, considering I had no experience in aviation, but I was open to it. "But," he said, "the only thing is that you'd have to close TAL Tours." I recognized that this new enterprise would require my full attention, but TAL had only become my business wholly a few years earlier, and I wasn't about to shut it down. I'd put too much into the company. I believed in it. It was successful. At this point, I was approaching forty and TAL was my professional legacy. Yet, here was a once-in-a-lifetime opportunity to take travel logistics to a whole other level.

"I'm not willing to close it," I said. "I'm willing to make it dormant." That was significant — I'd announce that it was being "paused," while I took on this new project, which I imagined would eventually be great for making new business contacts for when TAL emerged from hibernation. But I wasn't thinking like a businessman. I was thinking with my heart.

In hindsight, this was a smart move, but I can't give myself too much credit. Israir remains strong in Israel to this day.

But in the meantime, there was a five-year period when I was the US director of Israir.

Israir Airlines was founded in 1989 as Kanfei HaEmek, renaming itself with the catchier title of Israir in 1996. Their HQ is in Tel Aviv, their hub is Haifa Airport in Israel and, today, they have a boutique-sized fleet of eight planes flying to nineteen scheduled destinations. In recent years, they've expanded, becoming the second-largest Israeli airline, after El Al. I worked there from 2004 until 2008, overseeing its then-new charter service linking Israel with New York's JFK Airport. This became a regularly scheduled service in 2006, flying the Tel-Aviv to New York route.

The airline featured some elements that meant a lot to Jewish passengers. In 2007, it became the first airline to carry Torah scrolls on all flights, which passengers could use for prayer. We called them Sky-Torah scrolls. This led to more orthodox Jewish customers coming to us, particularly after dismay was expressed at El Al flying on Shabbat, the holy day in the Jewish week when everyone is meant to rest.

My main task was planning, opening, and running Israir's New York route, which also meant setting up everything about its business Stateside. I truly enjoyed it. Workwise, it was probably the most fun I've had. I did it all, from liaising with airports to negotiating catering contracts. Since we were new to the New York market, I came up with a marketing idea to offer $99 fares. That was the advertising pitch. Of course, $99 for a transatlantic flight is operating at a loss, so it was actually "fares from $99" with limited seats at that price (and middle seats), but it was a new tactic that paid off. These days it's common, but such a cheap transatlantic price was unheard of at the time.

We also had a homey touch. During the Jewish holidays, for instance, I'd bring kosher treats to the airport and personally hand them out to passengers. The emphasis was on familial informality. Other airlines had their staff wearing ties, while we wore polo shirts. I went with the tagline "Fun is in the air."

I enjoyed the free rein I was given, and the diversity of problems to solve. I dealt with landing contracts, catering, working with the pilots ... you name it.

Sometimes the business side was a little too homey. There was one moment when Israir had forgotten to pay a fuel bill on time. It was approaching Rosh Hashanah, the Jewish New Year, and this was the last flight that would get passengers home for the high holidays. JFK called me up and said, "What's the deal?" So I phoned my boss in Israel and said, "What's going on here?"

It was an honest mistake, a clerical error of some sort. He said, "Okay, we're going to take care of this right away." So they're back in Israel, trying to figure out how to wire the money to JFK, but it was Sunday and the banks were closed. We were stuck.

I start thinking on my feet. Filling a plane with fuel isn't a small operation. At the time, it cost around a hundred thousand dollars! So I'm running around the airport trying to see what I can do.

I found the person in charge of fueling and I joked, "Do you have self-serve?"

The guy looked at me and was trying to figure out if I was serious.

"Really," I continued. "Can I give you a credit card?"

Turns out it had never been done before, but they could do it.

"But, uh," the guy began after he'd calculated, "the bill would be $106,000."

I maxed out my credit cards, but got it done. Israir wired me the money the next day, but it was a wild experience. A story I've told many a time. As has the station manager at JFK, I imagine.

There was also an air accident during my tenure that others in the airline tried to cover up and didn't even tell me about. I learned when a *New York Times* reporter cold-called me and said, "Can you tell me about the accident?" I had to stop myself from instinctually replying, "What accident?"

I lied that I had the CEO of the airline on the other line, but I'd call her back.

I phoned the CEO and said, "What the heck is going on?" He said that he didn't really know, it had happened so recently.

He said, "You should say that you don't know anything."

"Okay," I replied. "But you know they're going to quote me on that. And that's not a good look."

I later learned that the accident had been two weeks prior, that Israir knew all about it, but had tried to cover it up. There I was, the US Director of the airline, and no one had told me a thing about it! This was prior to the social media revolution — today something like that couldn't remain a secret. The thing is, the passengers also didn't know how close they'd come to Armageddon.

It was just before 2 am on July 6, 2005. An Israir Boeing 767 plane, full with 262 passengers, accidentally taxied onto the wrong runway at JFK. It was foggy and rain hammered down. Visibility was low, but the pilots saw enough, as recorded on the flight tapes that were released by the Federal Aviation Administration a few weeks later, to shout, "Ground, Israir ... Ground, Ground, Israir ... Oh, he is taking off!"

The runway was occupied by a Douglas DC-8 cargo plane that was charging forward at full speed, prepared for takeoff. The Israir plane had somehow pulled up perpendicular to the occupied runway, with its nose sticking out across it. In a cinematic moment, the DC-8 managed to pull up in time and take off just over the Israir plane — the clearance between them was only forty-five feet!

The DC-8 pilot called to the control tower, "See that aircraft on runway twenty-two, right?"

"Did *you* see the aircraft?" the tower replied.

"I can't see a thing," the pilot retorted angrily.

Meanwhile, the Israir flight crew was also talking to the tower.

"Israir 102, are you clear?" the tower ground controller asked.

"We are now clear of the runway," came the Israir pilot's reply. "We crossed the runway."

"You *crossed* the runway!?"

"Affirmative. We crossed the runway by mistake."

Quite a mistake. Many airports at the time were equipped with an electronic gadget, ASDE-X, that would have sensed the two planes aiming for one another and prevented this long before it became a close call. But JFK didn't have it at the time. It was very nearly a disaster of epic proportions. But for me, as US representative of Israir, it was a public relations disaster already.

I'd handled everything in the US for Israir from the start, A to Z. I felt that it was my responsibility, and the airline's, to handle this, too. I was livid when I learned that the heads of Israir had tried to cover it up. I was ready to quit. I had also been completely excluded from the conversation.

So I called the reporter back and told her I'd talk to her but in person. That bought me 48 hours to figure out what I was going to say. I was able to gather more information, but I was furious.

I remained at Israir until they decided to close the transatlantic route. This was primarily due to the weakness of the dollar during the Recession of 2008.

In 2014, years after I'd left, they posted losses in the millions, and the company was being auctioned off in 2020. I was there for a brief period of great optimism, but their transatlantic flight program was short-lived.

The day the Israir owners told me they were shutting down the US office, August 5, 2008, was just about the worst day of my life. I'd poured everything into it. At least I had TAL Tours to return to. I'd brought much of the staff with me to Israir, so together we brought TAL out of hibernation. I was able to throw myself into it, which helped tremendously, keeping me from wallowing in upset. My old clients also came back. We'd kept in touch and they trusted me. I'm still grateful for the faith they put in me to resume our collaborations. Plus I'd made new connections and gained valuable experience in another aspect of the travel business.

Israir's difficulties unleashed my latent mental health issues. They'd been there all along — it wasn't because of a company failing — but it was the trigger for it.

Chapter 8

The Morally Questionable Misadventures of Travel Clients

Bangkok

Mental health is an invisible thing, but it touches all of us at some point or another. It's part of life.

— Kevin Love

It had been five years since I'd run a travel agency. But knowing I could reopen TAL Tours helped me bounce back and regain composure after having lost what was the professional highlight of my life to date: running an airline.

I wasn't sure where to begin, once TAL was back in operation. Fortunately, a handful of important clients from earlier days with TAL came back, as well as some new ones I'd developed during my airline tenure. They allowed TAL to be up and running within weeks, and I'm forever grateful to them for their support.

TAL's focus would be group travel, specializing in youth groups.

Specializing helps distinguish one agency from another. You need a lot of capital, advertising, and staff to be an all-rounder agency. Remaining boutique and specializing in a narrower slice of the market was an easier way to establish a foothold and a reputation.

I decided that TAL should hyperfocus on a) groups traveling as part of b) youth movements (like Bnei Akiva) with a c) Jewish focus, by guaranteeing kosher-compatible itineraries, while d) catering to luxury travelers. Dietary-specific tours might seem unusual and limiting, but there are plenty of people out there who keep strictly kosher but want to travel. Now, if you're traveling in the US or Israel, or to big cities like London or Paris, this isn't hard to do. But if you're keen to explore, say, Tibet or Tahiti, but need to keep kosher when it comes to all meals, both during transit and on location, then it can become a logistical adventure. That's when a quality tour company can really provide value to customers. You tell TAL Tours where you want to go, how many people, what your budget is and what your requirements are, and we sort out the rest.

We weren't aiming to be the highest-end tour agency, but I was prepared to turn business away if the budgets were below thresholds that I felt were feasible and made sense for us. I didn't want to turn business away, mind you. Newly up and running, I really needed any income we could muster. But at the end of the day, I didn't want to devote the same amount of time and energy for a $1,000 trip when I could arrange a $10,000 trip. The investment from my end would be the same. So I waited for the $10,000 trips and their like, hoping that I wouldn't regret passing on the smaller fry.

Most of our clients were not-for-profit groups who were happy to pay for quality service and locations. This doesn't mean five-star hotels, necessarily, but they knew I'd find them hotels of a certain level where they would be more than comfortable.

We were also extremely customer-focused. We would do right by the customer, no matter what. We often lost money, as a company if, for instance, a customer's flight came in late, and we needed to quickly book them on another one. Or I'd reimburse a customer from our own funds if an airline didn't reimburse them for, say, having lost their luggage. We'd swallow unexpected costs to keep the customer satisfied. I was able to make calls to do that because I was the one running everything. There was no one I had to report to, so I let my conscience guide me. I would imagine what I, as a potential customer, would be happiest with and I'd do that for our customers.

I also made my own personal availability a priority. I often joke that, if you write to me and I don't write you back, then I'm either on an airplane or dead. Well, I can't use the airplane excuse anymore since they all have free Wi-Fi. Although I don't like to speak on the phone, I'll answer right away. I'm especially efficient if you email or message me. I keep the phone calls to a minimum by requiring an appointment or asking a dedicated staff member to speak with you instead. This guarantees good service but also helps me with my neuroses about phone calls.

Even when I was lying in bed after a triple pulmonary embolism, I was in constant touch with clients. You may wonder if that triple pulmonary embolism was required *because* of my constant availability to clients, and I'm not sure I could argue that you were wrong. But part of my compulsive behavior is the need to please, to sort out, to respond to others, even to my own detriment. This makes for a neurotic, stressed, anxious me, but it makes for very satisfied customers. Happy customers brought me a sense of purpose and alleviated (if briefly) my own anxieties. It's a vicious circle, but one that leaves others pleased. After decades of this, I finally realized that I need to take care of myself, too. But for most of my life, tending to the wellbeing of others has been almost an obsession, certainly a soothing tendency that temporarily blanketed my anxiety ... until I wondered who I needed to tend to next.

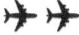

I'm in the service business, and I've had clients who were looking to be "serviced" in ways that extend beyond the magnet pole of my moral compass.

I was at a tourism trade show in Bangkok in the late '90s. The Cypriot Tourism Board paid my way, as they were hoping to open up a US-Cyprus flight route and wanted my input and assistance. I'm never going to say no to a free business-class plane ticket, so off I went. Israelis tend to find one another when abroad, and either become fast friends or, as happens more often, start arguing. I found myself there with an Israeli politician, among a group of Israelis at the event who wound up gravitating together. The politician was in Bangkok with a single goal in mind: sex. Prostitution is legal there, and Bangkok is a destination for "gentlemen" interested in partaking. Well, this politician was one such gentleman. I'm the exact opposite. The very idea freaks me out. Not my cup of tea. The idea of intimate contact with a stranger who has been having intimate contact with many other strangers throughout the day sounds like a nightmare to me.

But the politician, as a well-known figure, was the solar nexus of this group of Israeli trade show delegates. And he was there with his security team. We're walking through Bangkok, and he's got his bodyguards proactively seeking out prostitutes. I'm walking along, thinking, *Really? Is this what we vote for?* This was more than twenty years ago, and I was naïve then. Heck, I'm still naïve now. Evidence of my naivety is that this behavior from a well-known politician shocked me then and it would still shock me now, despite the overt evidence from many a politician that this should no longer be surprising. All I can remember thinking was, *Thank goodness he's not a TAL Tours customer, because then I'd have to be his prostitute provider, instead of his security staff.*

Once, in Ottawa in the early '90s, I prepared a conference for a Zionist organization. The keynote speaker was an important man who was both a former Israeli diplomat and the head of an important Jewish agency. I oversaw entertaining him. I went up to his hotel room to take him out to dinner. His security guard, who was standing in front of his room, told me to go on in. So in I went.

Turns out he wasn't alone, nor was he dressed. He didn't seem phased, but this was one of many formative traumas of my adult professional life.

Back at the start of TAL Tours, when the original partners were there, we had a lucrative deal representing the largest tourism company focused on the US and Israel. They were giving us all kinds of marketing money in sums unheard of at the time. It was early days for us, and we were happy to be the beneficiaries, and so wanted to keep these bread-and-butter clients pleased. They had us as their US presence and were providing enough income that we could set up a dedicated marketing team in our office.

Once the two guys who ran that company were in the US, and it was our job to entertain them. In my innocence, I figured that this meant we'd take them out for dinner. We did that, but they wanted to tour each of the cities where they'd be doing business. So we accompanied them on a fifteen-city grand tour of the US. Each location was full of meetings and seminars, and they'd wind up encountering hundreds of travel agents, either those with whom they already worked or agents who they hoped would add their travel packages to their agency offerings. It was a whirlwind, one night in each city.

But every night, they wanted to party.

I'm not a party person. But I had to take them out on the town, so they could sample the nightlife at every stop on the itinerary.

One night, when we were in Dallas, they heard about this bar in Fort Worth. I hate bars to begin with, and I'm not a fan of Fort Worth. So off we went, in my rental car. I was the designated driver.

We walked into the bar, and all the guys could talk about was a "Dancing table. We want dancing tables."

I didn't know what a dancing table was. I figured that it wasn't a table that dances. Maybe it was a table next to the stage, and we'd be taking in a tap dance performance? What did I know?

The two guys didn't speak perfect English, so it was my job to sort everything out. I went over to a staff member at the bar, and said, "Can we get a dancing table?" The staff member looked at me and started laughing.

"Table dancing. You want a table dance."

I didn't know what that was, either, but I found out. I still feel pretty traumatized by this incident. For the benefit of any readers who are at my epic level of naivety, table dancing is when mostly naked (or occasionally, I'm told, very naked) women come to your table and sort of dance around you in a sexually suggestive manner. You're supposed to buy these women overpriced drinks to encourage them to continue dancing in this sexually suggestive manner at your table, rather than at a neighboring one. You are also encouraged to place cash in, on, under, and around the scantily clad aspects of these women. As in, sliding a ten-dollar bill into the elastic waistband of their "undergarments."

You can imagine that this was my idea of a horror film. I was so uncomfortable that my body was locked into a sort of living rigor mortis. I remember a wash of ten-dollar bills splayed out on our table, with these ladies dancing around us, and my eyes were *locked* onto the bills, to the point that I still remember the serial numbers printed on some of them.

Needless to say, I've had my fair share of entertaining Israelis in weird ways.

Chapter 9

Where Does a Traveler Call Home?

Israel

I am not afraid of storms for I am learning how to sail my ship.

— **Amy March** in *Little Women*

For someone with three passports, who travels for more days of the year than he's in any one place, it's reasonable to ask how you choose where to call home. For me, the choice of eventually settling in Israel, after most of my life was spent in the US, is a surprise. Well, a surprise to someone who didn't come from a background similar to mine. Carol and I were "brainwashed" (in a good way) through Bnei Akiva to dream of emigrating to Israel. The dream remained but the logistics didn't line up for a long time. We were settled in the United States when our children arrived. That thought lingered — perhaps one day in Israel — but the time never felt right. We raised the kids with the dream intact, carrying on the benevolent brainwashing tradition of idealizing a move to the motherland, a homecoming to the land of our forefathers. The narrative was, "We've always wanted to do it but probably never will." Whether it was the biological clock or decades of creeping guilt at having ignored all that friendly brainwashing for so long, in our mid-forties, Carol and I decided that it was time. Or rather, that there would never be a perfect time, so we might as well do it now. When we mentioned this to the kids one evening over dinner, they turned to each other with smiles, and said, "Hey, I think they're serious this time."

We moved to Israel when I was aged forty-seven, fulfilling the Zionist drive of my youth. The surprise comes to those who knew that my early experiences with the country were entirely negative.

My first visit was when I was ten, in 1973. My paternal grandfather had died a year before, and my grandmother decided that it was time to take me and my brother there. Our flight over was turbulent, bouncing around in an old Boeing 707, and I was meeting family for the first time. There was much cheek-pinching (I was in a tubby phase, with my parents constantly reminding me of my weight), especially on the part of my numerous great-aunts. We didn't do much sightseeing, other than visiting the Western Wall in Jerusalem, the only remaining wall from the great Second Temple to survive the millennia, and a focal point for prayer.

We visited my grandfather's grave during the Jewish High Holidays period. A few weeks into the trip, the Yom Kippur War broke out. We made it onto the first flight back — a few days later, and we would've been stuck there, in a warzone. My association with Israel for many decades was as a nerve-wracking war zone full of people I didn't know trying to pinch my chubby cheeks in small, crowded apartments not much bigger than walk-in closets. If someone said, "Israel," I'd get nervous. I never wanted to go back. I was traumatized.

So how did I wind up calling it home and starting to love it?

My renewed interest in Israel came during my high school period working with Bnei Akiva. After 11th grade, I spent the summer at a Zionist camp. In addition to your average camp activities (swimming, bonfires with marshmallows), Camp Moshava promoted Judaism and Israel. The camp was such fun. This is what shifted my association with Israel from that early, upsetting trip to something positive. Everyone at the camp spoke glowingly of Israel as a place of welcome and possibility, a home for a people who have been in diaspora for millennia. Everyone was talking about going to Israel, not just for holidays but to move there, to the Jewish homeland. So I wasn't going to be the only one not to go.

I was planning to take a gap year between high school and college. Taking a year off wasn't done much at the time — almost everyone went straight on to university. But I opted to spend that year enrolled in a special program that involved getting in deeper touch with our Jewish heritage through travel. Thirteen of us journeyed through Eastern Europe, learning about the Holocaust, before the group expanded to forty to spend a year in Israel. To be honest, I was more excited about the social component than about Israel itself — many new friends of mine, made at camp, were among the teenagers attending. But this felt exciting. It was an early foundation for my passion for travel, but it also felt exotic and slightly subversive, since this was the Iron Curtain era, and you weren't really allowed to go to Eastern Europe. Through this program, we could visit places that were otherwise not welcoming.

The thirty-nine of us spent several weeks in Poland, Hungary, Austria, and Germany. We visited concentration camps. These days it's a requirement of the German school system to visit the camps, and many tourists go while on holiday. Back when we went, in 1980, no one visited them. We had to get special permission and the local authorities looked upon our group with suspicion. Government officials were constantly harassing us with questions — they just weren't used to student groups, especially from the United States and with an interest in Israel. This added a flair of danger to the proceedings. We were fresh out of high school, on a post-graduation high, away from home, independent, on top of the world — and also a little nervous that we'd end up thrown into a Polish prison. Those were the days of politically incorrect "Polish jokes," which we shared in whispers, afraid that a Polish policeman would overhear us, wondering, "How many Poles does it take to screw in a lightbulb," and reply with, "The same number that it takes to lock up teenage boys in jail."

We did silly, childish things but there was freedom to it. Once in Hungary, we got stuck in an elevator for hours, as we'd all climbed inside, and the elevator couldn't handle the weight. These were the sort of bonding experiences that endure — I'm still in touch with some of the friends from that trip to this day. Some are even my neighbors today.

It was a period of growth for me. We were learning about our heritage, as much about being human as about being Jewish. I'm a great proponent of early, extensive travel abroad, ideally where you must speak a foreign language.

TRAVEL THERAPY

It's the fastest way to mature, to build confidence and introspection.

Most of this trip was spent in Israel, and much of that on a kibbutz. A kibbutz is a social collective farming community. Families and individuals gathered on a patch of land to create a village situation, usually of no more than two-hundred individuals, with both social and economic sharing and equality. The idea was that no one owned anything: from tools to clothing to dishes to donations, it was all part of the kibbutz's common treasury. Meals were taken together in communal halls and even childcare was a group effort. A "differential wage" system was in place, in which each member of the kibbutz received an equal amount of the budget, regardless of the type of work they did there. Equality was evident in terms of gender, too.

The first kibbutz was established back in 1909, in Degania, in northern Israel. The concept is utopian, with aspects of socialism meeting Zionism. The practice really got going after 1927, when the United Kibbutz Movement was set up. Some settlements were more religious, others more interested in the social side. The socialist component was less of a factor by the time I was on a kibbutz. It was more of a village with communal elements, families living in their own residences, for instance, rather than a true socialist experiment. Back in the day, children lived together in special housing on the kibbutz, not exclusively with their parents.

It's still a major element of Israeli life. In 2010, there were 270 kibbutzim registered in Israel, with more than 120,000 people living in them. While originally agricultural, kibbutzim began to integrate industry and create products to the point where they accounted for 9% of Israel's industrial production — valued at some $8 billion a year, as well as a whopping 40% of Israel's agriculture, worth nearly $2 billion a year. One 200-member kibbutz, Kibbutz Sasa in Upper Galilee, functions like a live-in powerhouse business, with industrial facilities producing plastics for the military that earn a reported $850 million a year!

My experience was low-key and more experimental. Carol has long wanted to live on a kibbutz, even long-term. But I need my own space, and this is not a thing in kibbutz life. My experience was positive but for me, it had to be a finite one. I made good friends, and several of them happen to live near me today. My time there was divided, with half the day at work and half the day studying Hebrew and Judaism. I tried working in the fields, for example, picking oranges. Wasn't for me. I'm not an outdoor person, or at least I wasn't so at the time, so I did most of my work in the dining hall.

The eleven months on the kibbutz featured periodic field trips. One of them was to a man-made water slide, sort of like a homemade version of Six Flags. Everyone's sliding down it and having a great time. I got the brilliant idea to slide down headfirst, rather than feet first.

I don't remember the rest. I woke up back at the kibbutz's infirmary. One of my friends was an EMT and he'd leapt to my rescue. I'd managed to cut myself up pretty badly and get friction burns on my skin, head, and arms, I suppose from sand that was lurking on the manmade slide. I was roughed up enough that I couldn't do any work for a month.

Convalescing, I felt worthless. It's one thing to lay low at home, but if you're stuck in bed in the midst of a working collective, it feels worse. I'm also a capitalist, not a socialist, so the whole thing, while probably an enriching experience to try out, just wasn't for me. I need my space. I don't want everyone to know everything about what I'm doing. On a kibbutz, your fellow kibbutznik will know more about you than you know about you. That's what I pay a therapist for. A mentor of mine suggested that kibbutz life could be great, as you're directly contributing to society. I figure I can contribute to society while still having my own room I can retreat to when I feel the need.

Despite a few burns and the feeling that kibbutz life wasn't my cup of Carmel Wine, from that point on, I had a positive association with the country and thought that I might like to live there. This was cemented when I met Carol, as she also wanted to live in Israel. From our early days together, it was never a question of *if* we would move there, but of *when*. The logistics of life and work delayed our arrival, but never dissuaded us from it. We would only pick up and move when I was forty-seven and Carol was forty-five. It's hard to pick up and move then — you're settled into a rhythm; you've got a house and cars and kids in school with their friends. But if the dream and passion have always been there, then you find a way to fulfill them. I was speaking about the blessings of Israel so often for Bnei Akiva that they became self-evident to me. I grew more enthralled with Israel the more I spoke about it to others.

I began to visit often after that senior year high school trip. Visits in my early adulthood just felt very comfortable. That year abroad on the kibbutz had been positive. I'd made a great group of friends and I saw everything Israel had to offer. From that point on, I'd always wanted to live there. I didn't pick up and move like many of my friends did as soon as we were married, although that was our plan. With the job offer in New York, my move was postponed a long time. But the seed of desire was planted and usurped the negative feeling of my youth. Usurped but did not erase it. I made a conscious decision not to be cowed by my fear, especially when I saw so much benefit in living there.

My children grew up with my wife's and my enthusiasm. Our children knew we wanted to live there, but since they were raised in New York they didn't actually think we were going to move there. We visited Israel as a family during school vacations, and the kids went to summer camp in Israel. But when we did, it felt self-evident and was well-received by all.

When it came time to move to Israel, we had a few conditions that drove where we wanted to buy a home. It had to be near an airport, as I knew I'd be traveling a lot. It had to be near a gym. And it had to be near a dry cleaner, so I could get my shirts done. Not too much to ask, right? Well, two out of three ain't bad, as they say. We're now fifteen minutes from the airport. There's a gym right nearby, but I don't go to it — I prefer the one ten minutes away. No dry cleaner. So, you might think, you took to cleaning and ironing your own shirts, didn't you, Stuart? Nah. I fly my worn shirts to the US to be laundered. Yup. Look, I go so often, and I don't need a lot of dress shirts when I'm in Israel. So when I'm in the US, where there's a dry cleaner in every neighborhood, I bring them imported, dirty shirts.

We've only lived in one place in Israel: in a gated community, Hashmonaim, just outside the city of Modi'in. It's about twenty miles southeast of Tel Aviv and the same distance west of Jerusalem. The city is home to around 100,000 people and, historically, it's where the Maccabees were based. The Maccabees were a group of Jewish rebels who overthrew the invading Seleucid forces that were occupying Judea in the second century BCE. The story of their successful revolution is celebrated every year with the Jewish Hanukkah tradition. When we first arrived, we rented a home but by the second year we'd bought a home, and there we remain. Around half of the population of our neighborhood immigrated from the US or another anglophone country, so there's a touchstone of language and homecoming immigration, as I like to think of it, with those around us.

We wanted a house, rather than an apartment. My initial image of life in Israel, dating back fifty years from now, thirty-seven since we made the move, was visiting my relatives who lived in tiny, compact apartments. That wasn't for me. During my year abroad in Israel, I spent time on a kibbutz, a kind of collective socialist settlement where work and life are shared among a community. That also wasn't for me, though Carol really liked kibbutz life. I've always needed my space in a house where I can slip away and have some me-time. We managed to find a house that didn't sacrifice any of the conveniences that we'd gotten used to in the US, with plenty of room for guests. Best of all, we are part of a community of lovely, welcoming neighbors.

I sometimes look at the benefits of living in different countries and see that the cliché that the grass is always greener is there for a reason. We tend to focus on what could be better, wondering if the path not taken is the preferable one. Each person must make the judgment call for themselves.

For me, one of the key benefits of living in Israel over the US is socialized medicine. The quality of medical care in the US can be the best in the world, but you have to pay dearly for it, and most cannot afford it. In Israel, the national health service is solid and essentially free (though you do need to pay for the very best services, which remain private). That said, to see a specialist, you often need to wait a long time or have a "protekzia." This is a very Israeli term worth introducing.

Want to find a job in Israel or get the pothole in your street fixed? Sure, you might find employment by sending out a resumé or resolve your pothole situation by petitioning the city council, but the most direct route to success is often "protekzia," also known as "Vitamin P." Protekzia is all about protection, as it sounds, but not in that mafia-style "I won't break your windows anymore if you pay me protection money" way. It's a word that connotes the importance of connections, of having friends in the right places, and, sometimes, of blatant nepotism. It means that you know someone who can sort you out, do you a favor, and streamline the path to whatever you need.

The mental health care level in Israel is weak, as it has yet to be made a priority by the powers-that-be. It's one of my goals, and the goal of many others, to prioritize it, but it will be a long road. The first step is to shed the stigmas surrounding mental health. This isn't a policy issue but a social one, making it harder, less tangible, to work against. To this end, I helped start a project, deconstructingstigma.org, which has made initial strides. Aside from that, the cost of living in Israel is exceedingly high, as is the cost of food, though, of course, this depends on where you want to live and what you want to eat. But those sorts of cost-of-living comparisons don't tell the whole story.

In Israel, people live for today. Israelis aren't really about planning for tomorrow, looking to the future, long-term. They enjoy life in the moment in a way that I don't necessarily see in other countries, the US especially.

I'm still learning to be more Israeli in this sense. By now you'll know that living in the moment isn't really my personality trait. I'm always planning for the future: where my next paycheck will come from, how I'm going to afford this and that, where society as a whole is headed. Israelis are more "if you've got money, spend it." A true Israeli goes into overdraft at their bank with some regularity. An American would never dream of living beyond their credit line. I admire the "enjoy the moment" attitude, even if I can't fully get myself to commit to it.

Israelis are also extremely stubborn. This is a cliché, but it's a true one. This can be a good thing, and necessary for survival when surrounded by enemies, like when Israelis team together for a common cause. It can also be a not-so-good thing, like if you get into an argument with a neighbor over where your property lines run (just to clarify, this is purely hypothetical — my neighbors are lovely and have clearly defined property lines).

I'm a true Zionist, in love with Israel, but that doesn't mean that I don't see downsides. I've become disenchanted with the mental health system. There's far too much bureaucracy. Those complaints could be filed in any number of countries, of course. But the negatives have given me the motivation to try and do more to be part of the change that I'd like to see. I don't have the will to go and picket in front of the Knesset, the Israeli parliament. Not my style. I do what I can. For instance, launching the Deconstructing Stigma Project and Mental Health First Aid. These were projects to support the mental health system. We approached the government with them. They weren't interested. My attitude was, "We're doing this, with or without you." Governmental adoption would be far more broadly effective, but I'd rather do a little good than none.

I'm not sure my connection to Israel is particularly spiritual. I often feel more spiritually connected elsewhere. This is because, when I'm traveling, I feel that I'm an informal representative of Judaism and the Jewish people, so I'm more spiritually connected as a Jew when I'm away from Israel. Back home, if I visit the Western Wall or a holy city, I do feel a spiritual link to my ancestors. But I think it's a more forced connection because I know that I'm *supposed* to feel it when I'm in a place of collective prayer. I feel most spiritual when I'm volunteering abroad, representing Judaism and Israel by myself, just as Stuart Katz, not as part of an organization.

The biggest benefit for me is the fact that I call a Jewish state home — it's the geography and history, rather than the spiritual side. This is where Jews can feel at home. Historically, we've been a wandering people, and not by choice. It's not in our nature to conquer and colonize. Our military victories, dating back to Biblical times, have been in self-defense against invaders. We've long been marginalized and persecuted and had to make the best of the limits that nations and societies and empires have imposed on us, like being forced to live in ghettos or being disbarred from crafts and trades. Finally, the ancient home of the Jews is officially our home once more. And it feels like a homecoming to live here.

I've heard the same term over and over among immigrants to Israel. It's an emotional homecoming. It makes me think of my grandfather's family and other relatives who didn't leave Europe and perished in the Holocaust. The State of Israel was always going to be established, but it was established far more quickly because of the Holocaust. I feel living here is an opportunity, but also an obligation. Living here honors the memories of my relatives who were killed, of my people who that 1% of evil humans tried to literally erase from the planet. Israel as a state rises from those ashes. We have an opportunity to build here. We are the survivors. We are the architects and inhabitants of a Jewish state. But it's a state that welcomes anyone, of any religion, gender, you name it. I'm very proud of that and proud to be part of a country that does that. I hope we'll be able to continue in that direction in the future. To let Israel become a place of homecoming for anyone who wishes to call it home.

One of the major problems in Israel is that more than one cultural group considers parts of the country their homeland. This is a constant issue with Palestinians and Israelis particularly in the Gaza, Judea, and Samaria regions.

One chapter in my web of crisis volunteer work was at Sderot, a city of some 30,000 less than one mile from Gaza in Israel, originally founded in 1951 for newly arrived families from Iran and Kurdistan. The name means "boulevards" in Hebrew — a long road planted with eucalyptus trees runs through its center. and the roads through the settlement made international headlines when they were targeted by the Palestinian military, from 2001-

2008, in rocket attacks that killed thirteen people and wounded many more. The land itself has, shall we say, a complicated history. It had been the site of a Palestinian village, Najd, which was depopulated during the Arab-Israeli War in 1948. It was a diverse place — in the 1960s, it was nearly 90% Moroccan immigrants, the rest Kurds. In the '90s, many Soviet Jews moved here, as did Ethiopians. The population increased to the point that the village was made a city in 1996. The planting of eucalyptus trees provided a raw material that the residents could process, to stimulate employment. This village was part of a de-desertification campaign, reclaiming the desert by planting greenery. "Making the desert bloom" is a significant component of Zionism.

In the summer of 2014, I became involved in Tzuk Eitan, "Operation Protective Edge," as the 2014 Gaza War was also called. Sderot had been occupied by Israeli soldiers as part of the long-standing conflicts over the Gaza Strip, part of the so-called Second Intifada in 2001. When Israel disengaged from Gaza in 2005, rocket attacks increased, to the point that over fifty rockets per week were hammering down on Sderot during the Gaza War from December 2008 to January 2009. I was one of many volunteers helping both soldiers and civilians in the conflict zone. A rocket defense system, called Iron Dome, was installed, effectively intercepting incoming rockets, mitigating the damage. Operation Protective Edge made for a conflict zone crisis in my home country. The UN estimated that some 100,000 homes were destroyed or badly damaged, not to mention over 2,000 Gazans killed and more than 10,000 wounded (including over 3,000 children).

I could share hundreds of stories of the many special people we met during roughly nine eye-opening, tragic, and yet inspiring weeks of visits to Sderot. Some friends and I developed a close affinity with a particular segment of the population there. Many of its residents lived below the designated poverty line and had to contend with not only the tragedy of the rockets coming in from Gaza but also the daily burdens of hunger and deprivation.

We visited soldiers in the area but also stopped in at the homes of many city residents. For the soldiers, our hope was to give them moral support. To let them know that people care about what they're doing. And to bring them some better fare than military rations. We wanted to support the residents in a different way. They are living with nonstop trauma on their doorstep. Some feel that the government is betraying them. A sympathetic ear and some kind words are always welcome. We'd noticed how bare the city seemed during our initial visits and learned that the deserted streets were due to residents' fear of leaving their apartments. We would usually meet with families in their "safe room," if they had one, as they waited in fear of the next rocket. Most Israeli homes or apartment buildings have a "safe room," called a *mamad*. It might be a bunker in the basement or a reinforced room on each floor of a larger structure. It is a legal requirement that every apartment in Sderot has its own safe room.

We met the Cohn family (note that I've altered some names throughout this book to protect privacy), parents with eight children. They subsist on maybe $500 a month. When I first met them, they lived in a rundown two-bedroom apartment for the ten of them (plus one on the way). The father had been fired as a bus driver and never found another job. Over the nine-plus years that I've known them and periodically visited, they moved apartments many times, and some of the children have become drug addicts and moved out. They just don't seem to be able to right the ship of their lives.

Another gentleman is Moshe. He lives alone in a studio apartment and is blind. We bring him food whenever we can. Visitors are rare for him — he's lonely and loves to chat, so any time I go to visit, he's delighted, and we have long conversations. He's always wanting to give us blessings and it's difficult for us to leave — we're painfully aware that we might be the only company he'll see for weeks at a time.

We met the Schwartz family during a period of conflict in the region. One of their three children was born with severe eye problems, requiring many surgeries. We visited them numerous times, but they never wanted us to come into their apartment. Nothing wrong with that, but it was a bit unusual, as most of the people we visited would welcome us. We wound up raising money for their child's next eye surgery. After many visits, they finally invited us to their apartment. While there, I noticed that their refrigerator was completely empty. Ever since, we bring them groceries every time we visit.

As for the children of Sderot, attempts were made to operate summer camps for them, but the children wouldn't go, due to their parents' fear of a rocket being launched in their path.

Once the military operation ended and our boys returned home — though many other boys didn't, I felt that we couldn't just abandon the residents of Sderot. They were not an abstract concern, but real individuals whose lives truly mattered.

TRAVEL THERAPY

At the beginning of September 2014, I assisted in bringing thirty southern Israeli business owners to the New York and New Jersey area of the United States. There we held eight merchant shows in which they could sell their goods and help recoup some of their losses. Southern Israel had been bombarded by rockets launched from Gaza during that period. Sderot got the worst of it, but most of the south was under regular attack. Businesses suffered tremendously as customers stayed home, fearing for their safety. By September, the bombardments had ceased, but economic recovery was going to be an uphill battle.

This approach was something I'd helped with before. Colleagues and I had invited Israeli businesses to take on a fifty-three-city US tour back in 2006. This was a time when tourists, particularly Americans, stopped coming to Israel due to concerns about the intifada, popular uprisings of Palestinians in Israel's West Bank and Gaza Strip. Tourists worried that travel to Israel was unsafe at the time, and so businesses catering to tourists suffered. We figured that, if Americans weren't coming to Israel, perhaps we could bring some Israeli businesses to America, to help them recoup their losses. This was before I was living in Israel, but it felt like something we could do to help.

There's a famous pedestrian mall in Jerusalem, full of hundreds of shops, most of which cater to tourists, selling souvenirs and such. We first thought to invite Israeli businesses to one big show on Long Island, which might bring in 10,000 people. But since winter was a slow season for business anyway, we thought to expand the concept and make it a traveling, nationwide tour. We wound up putting together a tour of fifty-three cities, with some forty vendors participating. We offered a reasonable package that covered flights, hotels, meals, and transportation — sort of like a summer camp on wheels for a two-and-a-half-month period. They went from city to city, setting up their goods in synagogues, Jewish community centers, auditoriums, etc. Members of the local Jewish community would help promote each stop. They did a great deal of business, with over 25,000 people visiting the vendors during the trip. From that perspective, it was successful.

While it was a success, it was not without its share of arguing. The vendors would complain about each other: "This guy has a better location than I do, I want to be near the entrance." The vendors began to go rogue and bring in their own tables and set them up wherever they wanted, so it got a little chaotic. The organizers would politely say, "Guys, you can't do that," and then they'd start arguing with us! The "summer camp on wheels" began to feel like a kindergarten. We wound up having to hire some assistants, more like babysitters, to coordinate it all, because I was working myself sick.

But they sold extremely well, and, at the end, all the vendors returned to Israel happy. I guess I'm a glutton for punishment, because I helped organize a similar, though lower-key tour in 2014 — fewer vendors and locations only in the New York/New Jersey area. This was a good deal less stressful, and it proved a good way to help Israeli businesses.

But businesses start from a point of advantage. They might have good seasons and bad ones, but I was most interested in helping those who were truly in need. Those who had little to nothing.

While I was helping with the 2014 mini-tour, someone asked me what my next project would be, since the war was over, and business should be returning to normal. It dawned on me that, for the people in the south of Israel — particularly in Sderot, which was at the fore of my mind — relief from the barrage of rockets only meant returning to a "normal" that included the struggle to put food on the table.

I decided then and there that I would continue to go to Sderot every week and help the residents to make ends meet. Ever since 2014, and still to this day, I go there most Fridays when I'm in Israel. I've kept this promise to myself, going to Sderot, either solo or with whatever friends or guests want to join. Before the visit, I would stop at four or five stores — a few of the local "makolet" (minimarts), a bakery, a fruit store, a candy store, a takeout joint — and buy food for between five and ten households. I found that older, single people prefer a prepared takeout meal, while families preferred bags of groceries. Once we arrived, Rav Pizem, the chief rabbi of Chabad Sderot, would accompany us as we delivered the food. Having been there about thirty-six years, this kind man understood the needs of Sderot's neediest citizens.

It was important to me not to be some anonymous delivery program, as is the most common approach elsewhere, to preserve the dignity of the recipients. We actually met with the recipients, talked with them, and found out about how their week went and, more importantly, what their needs were. There were some 300 families on the distribution list and more that were in need. Each week we reached up to ten of these families. It was all we could afford to donate, in time and money, and it felt like a drop in the ocean. But it's better to do a little, to do all you can, than nothing at all.

TRAVEL THERAPY

There were at least 150 kids I knew of in Sderot — perhaps more — who wanted to attend summer camps the following year but couldn't afford to. Their families struggled just to make ends meet. For me, it was important that these families and children were not an abstract concern but people we knew.

I asked a family we were visiting what the kids were doing during the summer. Their reply: "What else can they do? They'll be at home." When I asked the next family the same question, I received the same response. My next move formed swiftly in my mind.

My fellow volunteers and I wound up launching a charitable campaign to cover the basic expenses of sending some of these children from conflict zones to enjoy summer camp in which 350 kids engaged in sports, baking, field trips, and the like. When others heard what we were doing, they wanted to be a part of it. Some were so enthusiastic that they wanted to go with me on one of my trips there, while others would send food, both homemade and purchased, or clothes, games for children–whatever they needed. My friends and neighbors opened up their hearts and provided what assistance they could. To let those kids be kids, even while their homes were under constant threat of bombardment.

Chapter 10

Back Home as a Foreigner

Long Island

The man who moves a mountain begins by carrying away small stones.

— **Confucius**

When I lived in the US, I was always arranging missions to go to Israel and help out there in a time of need. Now, living in Israel, when I saw that former neighbors in the US needed assistance, I felt an obligation to do what I could. After having lived in the Five Towns of Long Island for many years, I came back to lend a hand in the wake of Hurricane Sandy.

Sandy was a hugely destructive Atlantic hurricane, the largest on record by diameter, with storm-force, Category three winds blasting a swath 1150 miles across. 233 people were killed in eight countries, causing over $70 billion in damage. What began as a tropical wave in the Caribbean Sea on October 22, 2012, within six hours had mounted into a Tropical Storm. Two days later it erupted into full hurricane force. Twenty-four states in the US were affected (amounting to $65 billion of the $70 billion in damage and

157 of the fatalities), but the worst of it struck New York and New Jersey, including Long Island. In New York, the airports were closed, as were all the subways and mass transits. The Brooklyn-Battery tunnel was one of seven that would be completely flooded, and the East River overflowed its banks, submerging parts of Lower Manhattan. Memories of Hurricane Irene, just a year before, were fresh. Coastlines were evacuated on October 29. Power was out on Halloween to six million people in fifteen states, including two million in New York. More than ten billion gallons of raw or only partially treated sewage erupted into the waters of New York and New Jersey. In the Chelsea neighborhood of Manhattan, a building's entire façade broke off, leaving the interior apartments open to the elements. New York State's damages were estimated at $42 billion. More than 100,000 homes on Long Island were severely damaged, with 2,000 entirely uninhabitable.

I tracked this from our new home in Israel. It particularly moved our family, since not long ago we had lived right in the path of the storm — many of our neighbors and friends suffered significant damage to their homes. Had we not emigrated to Israel, we would have been among those whose lives were in ruins. So much in life is a matter of timing and of seemingly separate threads coming together at an opportune moment. The genesis of a journey of volunteer work, returning to Long Island to do what we could to help, was an unlikely combination of a daughter's wish, the spark of new war activity in Israel, and a hurricane striking an ocean away. I would spend a week in New York, with six Israeli teens, there both to lend a hand in rebuilding efforts and as young ambassadors for Israel.

I first flew to volunteer on my own. Having once lived on Long Island, I had the same impulse to help out my former hometown areas as I had to help out Israel in times of crisis — it's a dual loyalty many of us have. Although I am now based on the other side of the Atlantic, the compulsion to help remains strong.

When I returned home to Hashmonaim after my week's sojourn, my youngest daughter was struck by the stories I told of the situation I found in the tri-state area, as well as the need for further assistance. Dafna, a teen at the time, was clearly ready to hop onto the next plane stateside with me and lend a hand herself. After some discussion, we reached a compromise: if she would wait until her school vacation, during Hanukkah, I would take her to the US with me if there was still a need for assistance.

So the deal was struck, and Dafna's enthusiasm spread to several of her friends, who also wanted to get involved. And so *Masa Hashemesh* was born. The requirements to become a member of this effort were simple. A willingness to give up a large part of one's holiday break, work from morning to night for an entire week, and pay one's own way.

We limited the trip to six teens, and I made certain that I either knew each kid or got to know them well enough to ensure that they would be a "good fit" for this volunteer crew.

We came up with an official name for our group because of my experience contacting various organizations in the US about volunteering. Invariably, they wanted to know with which organization I was affiliated. As we were strictly grassroots in our efforts, we decided to call ourselves *Masa Hashemesh* and create some semblance of being an official group. The name, which can be roughly translated to "Sunlight Journey," was selected with some thought, reflecting our desire to bring some sunshine to the areas we visited – particularly fitting during Hanukkah's season of light.

My years in the travel industry were put to good use, as I was able to quickly fit together an itinerary, make travel arrangements, find host homes, and iron out details to make the trip a meaningful one for both the group and those with whom we came in contact. In designing the trip itinerary, it was important that we achieve a balance of hands-on volunteer efforts to benefit the New York area, opportunities to represent Israel well among young Americans, and seasonal and social activities – after all, hard-working volunteers need time for relaxation and celebration.

What had started out as a simple plan for post-Sandy clean-up evolved into its larger mission when Israel once again found itself in armed conflict with Gaza. We decided that part of our mission should be to share information about Israel's situation with others and to emphasize the mutual support upon which our two countries both relied. Student to student dialogue seemed an ideal way to proceed with this mission.

So Masa Hashemesh moved forward with a critical underlying message: after decades of looking to the US for support, Israel also stands ready to offer its support to Americans, regardless of religion or ethnicity.

Our group landed in the United States and began its whirlwind week of demolition work, soup kitchens, school presentations, and holiday fellowship. Hurricane help would indeed involve a whirlwind of activities.

Our first day was a Thursday, December 6, when met at our hosts' homes, shortly after our arrival. We then began a day of visits with various youth organizations and schools.

At each stop, our group members shared their personal stories of life in Israel, answered questions, and encouraged their peers to become more involved in advocacy for Israel. Given that we had a group of healthy, hungry teens, we made time for dinner and a coffee shop visit in Plainview to end our first day. I'm a specialist at kosher holidays, so we were pleased to find a kosher pizza parlor as a spot to refuel.

After a full working Friday, we headed to Riverdale to prepare for Shabbat. Our Friday night dinner was hosted by an area family, with Bnei Akiva youth attending. This wonderful organization models itself on the principles of *aliyah*, love of the Jewish people, and love of Israel, and our group immediately felt at home. Dinner was followed by an *Oneg Shabbat*, a traditional gathering after the Friday night dinner, at the local synagogue. during which our group led discussions about what it's like to live as a teen in Israel today.

Shabbat (Saturday) included further interaction with the local teens, beginning with a teen *minyan* (a minimum of ten male congregants who are considered adults since they've had a Bar Mitzvah celebration) and concluding with *havdalah*, the ceremony at the end of the Sabbath. For the younger kids, the girls prepared a presentation on Hanukkah and life in Israel. A kiddush lunch followed and then we just relaxed with local teens in the teen lounge.

At 5:30 pm, we lit candles to commemorate the first night of Hanukkah. We then loaded our van and headed to Far Rockaway to celebrate with the local Young Israel of Long Beach synagogue, strengthening the light there in these devastated areas with our Israeli spirit (as manifested in song and dance). From here, we journeyed to yet another Hanukkah Party at the Young Israel of Brighton Beach. Their building was severely damaged during the hurricane, but we did our best to brighten the scene. It felt kind of cool that we were coming from the location of the miracle of Hanukkah (Hashmonaim) and bringing so much light to so many.

The time of year in which our trip occurred only heightened its significance to all who participated. It was particularly joyful to bring the Hanukkah spirit to many area residents who survived the hurricane. Our Saturday night celebrations in Long Beach and Brighton Beach were especially poignant. Although we were surrounded by the devastation of the recent storm, the evening gave testament to the survival skills of those who had been most affected. Our group was thrilled to be able to celebrate the season with them.

On Sunday, we spent several hours in Long Beach doing clean-up. As in the Arverne area, we were struck by how much damage was still visible, even seven weeks after the initial devastation wrought by Sandy. Our main project in Long Beach was to clean up the communal backyard and driveway of a condominium unit. The groups cheerfully removed piles of debris, even in the midst of a downpour. After the cleanup activity, we walked what was once the Long Beach boardwalk and had time to shiver on the beach before hightailing it back to a warmer location.

That afternoon we headed to Cedarhurst to visit with the Jewish Community Center (JCC) of the Five Towns Teen Program. Then our teens were given an evening on their own, which allowed them to visit with friends and relatives, or even catch a basketball game.

Monday was a very full day, starting in Brooklyn at St. John's Episcopal Church. At its Fort Hamilton Kitchen, we helped in the soup kitchen. Our task was to prepare fruits and vegetables and set tables for lunch. The soup kitchen had been set up by "Occupy Sandy" specifically to help those in need after the storm. My own culinary skills improved after cutting my share of tomatoes. We also engaged in extensive potato peeling and the of making egg salad and peanut butter and jelly sandwiches, feeding a few thousand people. We deliberately chose a Christian church as a locale, as it was important to help all people, regardless of faith or religion, and to represent Israel proudly in doing so.

Monday afternoon was filled with visits with students from several area high schools. After so much productive time spent chopping vegetables and giving presentations, the group enjoyed a Hanukkah party at our friends' home in North Woodmere.

Tuesday's itinerary included more school visits, in Lake Success and Brooklyn. As always, we shared stories from Israel and showed an inspirational video that the group put together prior to the trip. The day ended with a lovely Hanukkah dinner at Congregation Beth Sholom in Lawrence. It was sponsored by Jewish Community Center and Jewish Education Program in support of children with special needs and individuals who had been impacted by Sandy.

Our final day included visits to two more high schools. By mid-afternoon, we had completed our last presentation and headed to the airport for the long trip home. Then it was time for reflection on what we had experienced and its potential impact. In a total of six days, our small group had provided hands-on assistance in Sandy clean-up efforts in two locations (Arverne and Long Beach), prepared food for a local soup kitchen for survivors of Hurricane Sandy, and made presentations at over twenty gatherings of primarily students.

In addition to all the hard work, the group found a unique way to celebrate Hanukkah through overseas volunteerism. As one of these wonderful tenth graders told me, this Hanukkah was one of their best and most miraculous. For me, it was special not only because I was moved that Dafna wanted to join me on a volunteer mission, but also to see young people so earnest and determined to help. It was their initiative, not mine.

We helped with post-Sandy relief efforts, but more importantly, we shared an important message about our homeland. These six teens demonstrated that youth in Israel are no different from those in the US. They succeeded in de-mystifying Israel for curious youngsters in the United States, showing that Israel is a worthy ally and a great place to visit (or to live). It was a frequent point of interest to American teens that we had decided to live in Israel. All of the teens on the trip had either lived in the US previously or had parents who had lived there. It was a turbulent time for Israel, frequently in the news due to the conflicts and terrorist attacks, so the American students found it fascinating that we actually preferred to live there than in the US.

Students had many questions about Operation Pillar of Defense — Jews and non-Jews, public school and Yeshiva students alike were curious. This had recently been in the news. On November 14, 2012, the Israeli Defense Forces (IDF) launched a mission against Hamas, which had been bombarding the Gaza Strip with rockets. Hamas had also kidnapped and held Israeli soldier Gilad Shalit back in 2006 and only released him as part of a prisoner exchange in 2011. The IDF managed to eliminate Ahmed Jabari, second in command of the military wing of Hamas, in a targeted, precision airstrike. It was part of an eight-day offensive that hit more than 1,500 terrorist sites in the Gaza Strip. Hamas ordered their own civilians to be used as human shields, while targeting Israeli schools, homes, and even mosques across the border, showering Israel with more than 1,500 rockets. Nine hundred struck their targets, but hundreds were intercepted by Iron Dome batteries, which shot them down before they could strike. Six Israelis were killed and 240 wounded. It was the latest in the sad story of blood in the Gaza Strip. But hearing a bit about this on the evening news, or reading cold, hard numbers of wounded, do little to convey the real damage, the human loss. It hits home more and is easier to sympathize with people affected by the fighting. And so hearing directly from Israelis, teens at that, speaking from the heart and during a time when, with problems of their own back home, they chose to spend their limited holidays volunteering abroad — it was moving for all.

People also marveled that kids who might understandably feel vulnerable to attack felt a need to come and help others. I hope we put the security concerns about Israel in a more realistic perspective, as our teens assured others that they are not walking around afraid all the time, and that Israel remains a great place to visit. Several students even said they would like to visit Israel, which would not have been the case before our trip.

There were many misconceptions about Israel initially. Some of them were amusing. Kids were asked if they lived in tents and rode camels (no, that was *not* a joke). Normalizing people or other countries is the first step in acceptance and then support. By sharing their love of Israel, while showing they are just normal teens, our Masa Hashemesh project accomplished more than the best public relations firm could have.

Speaking of PR, our kids emphasized to their peers that they can also be advocates for Israel, via social media such as Facebook or Twitter, by telling the truth about our country. They offered to continue to educate their new friends whenever there was a question — and they're all Facebook friends now.

Everywhere our team worked, whether in a soup kitchen, demolition site, or classroom, people seemed genuinely impressed with the group's compassion, teamwork, and sense of purpose. They truly made a "Sunlight Journey" to America, sharing a little Israeli warmth and light along the way.

Recalling this, Dafna told me, "Growing up traveling was fun. Now I realize that traveling also has a purpose. The best antidepressant out there."

Chapter 11

A Trip with Each Child

Airport Lounges with My Children

If it is a virtue to love my neighbor as a human being, it must be a virtue — and not a vice — to love myself, since I am a human being too. There is no concept of man in which I myself am not included.

— Erich Fromm

In 2018, I surprised Carol. I remembered that she'd once forwarded me a social media post about the Panda Reserve in Chengdu, China. You can go to the reserve, see pandas in action, and even get a photo hugging one. (It's a quick hug, because pandas technically are bears, even if they prefer nibbling bamboo to mauling Panamanian-American-Israeli tourists). You must understand that Carol is totally trusting and easygoing. She'll let me take her on a trip without bothering with exactly how we're getting there, or even where we're going. She knows I'll sort it out, and she's generally happy to come along for the ride.

So I asked her if she'd be up for flying on the inaugural flight from Hong Kong to Tel Aviv on the airline Cathay Pacific. We'd been to Hong

Kong several times before, but I told her we could visit some other parts of China, like Ningbo, one of the country's oldest cities. She was up for it.

Off we went ahead of the inaugural, which would be the return flight for us. We flew from Tel Aviv to Amman, then on to Abu Dhabi, and finally to Hong Kong, before catching a flight to mainland China. With a six-hour layover in Hong Kong, I had just enough time to zip off and get measured for a tailor-made suit, which I'd pick up on our return.

Carol's thinking that we're off to Ningbo. I was carrying the tickets and Carol was cruising along through the airport beside me. We take a seat in a departure lounge with "Chengdu" clearly written as the destination. Carol doesn't seem to notice.

We board the plane, and the announcements are in Chinese. Carol's tuned out anyway, in the Zen zone of the experienced traveler in the company of someone else who's worrying about the details.

We land in China, deplane, and walk past various signs that read "Welcome to Chengdu," with posters of pandas everywhere. Carol is messaging our family WhatsApp group, writing "We just landed in Ningbo." I thought that this was hilarious, which encouraged the kids to play along, messaging back asking what we were going to see there. Off we went to our hotel, which even had the word Chengdu in its name. Carol still thinks we're in Ningbo.

The next day, a tour guide shows up. He doesn't really speak English but welcomes us into his car. We drive for about an hour and get out in front of a giant sign: "Chengdu Panda Reserve."

"Stuart, where are we?"

"At the Panda Reserve," I replied. "Remember when you forwarded me a link to it, like, two years ago?"

This was the first time she realized that we weren't in Ningbo.

In we went and had a great time. We even got photos next to a panda. I like my photo so much I use it as my profile picture.

I've traveled countless times one-on-one with Carol. I figured it would be good to have the same experience with each of my kids.

I decided to gift each of my four children with a one-to-one bonding trip to a place of their choice. This has been a wonderful creator of memories and a chance to spend quality time with each child — a very different dynamic from the pleasures (and occasional trials) of the full Katz family experience.

I've managed to go with all but my youngest, Dafna, but that trip is in the works.

My kids have consistently enthused about a Katz family practice which we called The Game. While that sounds somewhat sinister (possibly like a Michael Douglas movie), it was great fun. The short version: for many family trips, we wouldn't tell the kids, right off the bat, where we were going. We would make them guess and provide clues along the way, as we prepared for the trip. Each trip, and each rendition of The Game, was different. We'd make up clues that usually encouraged the kids to learn some geography. As they grew, we made the clues age-appropriate, more complex. In retrospect, I can't believe the number of hours that I actually spent on this, definitely far more than on the trip itself. Several times my kids refer to this game, which clearly made a good impression. It's also something that any parent could try out.

To give you a sense of what The Game entailed, here are some actual clues given, one a day, before we set off from New York. See if you can guess where we went. Hint: It was a multi-stop holiday with a theme of canals. (The answer is at the end of this chapter).

1. Train to the Plane
2. Across the Pond
3. Best Lounge at JFK
4. Time to Revive
5. Tulips by the Canal
6. You Visited Her Birthplace Now See Her Home
7. Eva
8. Canal by the Ghetto
9. Spaghetti, Tortellini, Pizza
10. Large Uncle
11. It's Good to Have Lots of Pounds
12. The Queen is Delighted We're Coming
13. You Say Soccer ... I Say Futbol
14. Tube It To M&S
15. Wilma Under the Sun
16. Se Habla Espanol
17. On the Canal
18. Birthplace of Someone Very Important

19.   Our Last Stop. Passport Still Required
20.   Nananana But with A "P"

We tend to plan ahead, as parents, and prep our kids to look forward to a trip. The only common surprise trip is to wake your kids in the small hours and tell them to quickly pack because you're off to Disney World. But if knowing about holidays in advance is the norm and we invert this occasionally (or even just once, no need to go "Full Katz" and play The Game around most of your holidays), then it will really stick in the kids' memories.

Because my children are wonderfully eloquent, rather than rewrite the stories they told me when I asked them about travel as a family in general, I've decided to leave it mostly in their own words.

ADINA

I have various memories of our trips, but one that really sticks out to me is our roots family trip to Eastern Europe. I'm so fortunate to have been to places that people only read about or see in Pinterest images. But this trip I remember as being such fun.

Growing up, we didn't take long family drives too often (which I am totally fine with), but something nice on this trip was that we did have long drives together. Also, the trip itself was a lot of fun, and I remember being very surprised by that, at the time. In hindsight, I think that we all knew (subconsciously or consciously) that it was a heavier topic trip, and we did our best to bring the good out of it.

We traveled to the concentration camp, Mauthausen, in which Great-Grandpa was held as a prisoner. It was surreal and sad to walk where Grandpa's father had — he made it out, but he didn't live much longer — he died shortly after he was liberated by the Allies. The visit made me even more grateful to have Grandpa at all. It was a tough trip psychologically because of what we were seeing, but one that produced a proper change in me. A trip that augmented my gratitude and appreciation for what I have. What we all have.

I've thought a lot about my attitude towards travel both pre- and post-Covid pandemic. As a young adult, I was aware that I had traveled to ten times the number of destinations that anyone dreams of in a lifetime. A part of me sometimes worries if I'll get to travel as an adult at all. Being a full-time working mom doesn't leave much room for that. Plus, if I'm honest, I'm a little nervous about traveling to unknown-to-me places with tiny toddlers. I have much respect for you and Mommy as parents in general, but specifically when it comes to travel, I have no idea how you did it. And sorry that I was a brat until I grew up a bit.

Having a father in the travel business and traveling for a significant percentage of each year had positive and negative sides to it. I've gone through different feelings about this. As a young child, my feelings were "Wow, why is everyone in my class's father a lawyer, doctor, or property manager? Mine is different and cool." As I got older, I didn't love when you were away as much. It meant being away for any amount of time and coming back tired. Now, at this point in my life, I can say that I truly admire you for doing what you love, for making a career out of it, as well as serving the world.

I really struggled as a teenager living in the Five Towns on Long Island. Even today, I still have such sad and negative memories of the girls in my classes. I do believe it's made me who I am today, and while I'm pretty extroverted, I can pick out people who seem less comfortable and I try to reach out to them first.

For our one-on-one trip together, it was my senior year of high school. I was seventeen and I had my driving test scheduled. You asked if I wanted to go with you to Hawaii and I was more than happy to push off my test (who knew I'd only get my driver's license eight years later and in another country?) At that age, parents and kids aren't always in sync, but you were understanding of that. We did our own things during the day and reconvened each evening. We were similar and compatible as travel buddies. Giving me the freedom to explore on my own during the day made me look forward to getting together at night.

ILAN

Growing up, I most enjoyed the cruises. There's something special about being secluded, away from civilization, but with lots of fun things to do. This combination made me happy. The trips I remember most vividly were those that involved attending sporting events. Football games in Saint Louis, San Antonio, Houston, Phoenix, and the national championship in Dallas. And when Petco Park opened in San Diego, we went to a Padres game. My least favorite aspect? When stress got the best of us.

In retrospect, I can now say that I definitely took for granted how much I got to travel the world as a kid. How lucky I was growing up and only realized it later! Now that our family has expanded, I have a special appreciation for travel, and how much we got to do.

Of all the places we lived, the one that stands out was North Woodmere, in the Five Towns area of Long Island. It was where I was home for the longest and all of my childhood memories were there. It's funny because I loved it there, but Adina hated it. Same place, same family, totally different experiences.

The most special trip of all was when we went to Chile. It was special to go just with you. It made me feel important. You had a business meeting in Chile, but it's funny, I was proud to go with you. I know that our plane got diverted to some random, small airport in Mendoza, Argentina. We watched the movie "Old School" together on the plane. Another thought has stuck with me: I accompanied you to a business meeting in a hotel and I was so surprised that you didn't order Diet Coke with ice.

Like any sports junkie, I loved to attend sporting events. Just about anything other than golf. I loved the several times we did March Madness trips, visiting NCAA college basketball games, while adding in the odd baseball or football game, if it was on our route. The first NCAA trip I remember was when we spent time in San Antonio and St. Louis. The games in San Antonio are still vivid memories. Both were one-point games at the Alamo Dome, which was massive. We spent Shabbat in St. Louis and ate lunch at the rabbi's house. I played with his son, who was really energetic. We didn't have as good seats at the Elite 8 game on the following Sunday, but Florida beat Oregon on their way to the Championship.

The next year we went to Phoenix and Houston. That Shabbat in Houston is also a strong memory. I remember being captivated by the son of one of your friends there, playing a basketball video game with Rockets players. The game that Sunday was Houston against Memphis. The massive stadium in Houston was filled with burnt orange, except for a sliver of Memphis blue.

Derrick Rose of the Rockets put on the single greatest performance I can remember witnessing in a basketball game to this day.

I'm not sure that any one trip deepened our relationship — it was already deep — but our sports trips were amazing experiences and it's good that we did them when I was old enough to appreciate how truly fortunate I was.

GILAD

The first thing to mention is that my memory has never been as good as yours, nor have I documented things as well. So some trips I remember either not as well, or differently. I suppose that's the purpose of your writing project, to gather what bits of memory we can. I'm not sure I recall our first family trip. I have some bits and pieces in mind, like when we first flew to Israel. Dafna and you and Mommy sat in First Class on the 747 and watched "The Hunchback of Notre Dame," while the three of us other kids sat in coach. We were fine with that, having fun in the back.

The first trip I remember clearly was Thailand and Hong Kong. It was right after Bubbie died, Mom's grandmother, in 2004 — aged 106, supposedly, though we were never quite sure. Let's say she was 106. We went to the funeral, then to Baltimore for a family reunion, before heading off on a weeklong family trip. We started the trip in Dallas but there were connections we didn't expect, and some of us started crying because you had to get on another plane for a trip to Tokyo without us. What I remember most regularly were the delays on our trips.

The way you and Mommy planned trips were a few days here and there, then off again. We'd take one or two local tours each day to see the sites. I don't do tours like that anymore, but I liked them then. They do offer more impact because you see the sites with local guides, instead of drifting as tourists. But I feel like it can take away from the overall experience of just being in a new place.

We were in Bangkok just before the big tsunami. You, me, and Dafna went out to a 7-11 — I was surprised to find a 7-11 there. Back then I found wandering places, visiting markets, and such, kind of boring, but they were on your checklists of what to do. That was before the internet was so easily accessible, so it made sense to organize ahead of time. You are a tour operator, after all.

I also remember the New Orleans trip, by cruise ship. That was a positive experience, though I don't like cruise ships today.

It's funny, but I don't remember what I disliked about trips. In general, for me, I gloss over anything bad and don't recall it. That's a good thing, I think. I do remember fighting with Ilan or disagreeing with what he wanted to do.

I always loved traveling growing up. I still do, particularly adventure travel, and I think that's because I'm comfortable with it. The last time I was in Hanoi, Vietnam I recognized places, even though it was twenty years ago that I was last there. But back then I was riding along with you in the lead. Today I'm surprised to see how much everything costs — money wasn't a factor as a kid, since you took care of everything for us. This has changed my attitude to travel and my appreciation for all you did for us. When I backpacked for a year, I spent over $15,000, including flying lessons and stuff like that. An awareness of the cost of travel changes things, the shift from passive child to planning adult.

It made a big difference for me growing up with a father in the travel industry. Back then I just saw it as my father's job, but a particularly cool one. Other kids' parents were doctors, lawyers, whatever, and they lived pretty cookie-cutter existences. And a fair number of people live their lives as their parents did. My friends all did. They grew up on Long Island, went to law school, then returned to the New York/New Jersey area. They had a consistency to their lives, maybe a predictability, that we didn't have: New York suburbs, nice facades, PlayStations, totally American. I got a PSP PlayStation when I got my driver's license, years after my peers, but I was content with that because we had other experiences.

I'm trying to remember how old I was when I found what was different about our lives valuable. I can't remember if it was Ilan or Adina but one time, we were talking about how it was cool that we didn't just go to the Caribbean or Miami, like everyone else on holiday, but we got to travel the world and experience new things, from business class flights to lounges and whatever other benefits came with your work.

The earliest travel-related memory I have was when I was probably five or so. You had a bunch of weekly meetings in DC and brought me with you, flying out of Reagan Airport. Our first trip alone together. It was almost every Sunday for a period of time, over to the business lounge, then off you'd go. I spent a lot of time at that airport or at your office, more than my siblings. I appreciated that you'd bring me with you. It enhanced my love for travel.

I particularly recall coming to Israel with you, maybe November 2003. We came for just Thanksgiving weekend, and we went to a burger bar for the first time.

Our bigger trip alone together was to Germany and England. We went to Big Ben and Buckingham Palace the week that the Queen Mother died — it came rushing back when I was in England when the Queen herself died now, in 2022. That was a big step for me because it was my first trip to another country. It was the beginning of my travel life, which continues and grows today. That's also when I started my collection. I still collect cans, a habit that began collecting soda cans from around the world as a kid. It began when you took me, aged seven or so, with a group of rabbis to Germany. You were busy with grownup stuff, trying to open dialogues between rabbinical communities in the US and Germany. I was busy collecting soda cans.

DAFNA

I recall the games we used to play when on the road, especially the game of finding out where we were traveling to. Sometimes we found out all the places we were going beforehand. But it was magical to sometimes get somewhere, thinking we've finally traveled long enough, only for you to surprise us with the news that we were only transferring *through* there. My most-quoted line? "Another plane?"

It was great that you made a guessing game out of it. We'd have papers across the house hanging on the wall with lists of cities or countries, and we'd get hints and slowly begin to cross the cities out until we found out where we were going.

Some of the clues were different for each of us kids. For example, I remember getting a doll as a clue, when I was a little girl. Gilad would get some sort of foreign currency.

During the trips, we would also get super fun surprises. Once we were supposed to drive from North to South Dakota in two separate cars. We were bummed that we weren't going to be all together, although I decided to go in your car, thanks to the promise of a visit to the Jelly Belly jellybean factory (sorry team Mommy — on a previous trip to California Mom's car had gotten lost, and only your car made it to the factory, so I was hedging my bets). Outside our hotel, we waited for you guys to come with the cars that you had both gone to get. Then around the bend you came — in a limo! We were thrilled that we would all be together. Okay, maybe we were also thrilled because we could all drink all the Diet Coke we wanted in the limo. Either way, it was super memorable.

We went to British Columbia on a ferry and thought we were going back that way, too. That is until we arrived at the port and a seaplane was waiting for us! We were so surprised. We were less surprised when Gilad started touching all the buttons, asking what they did, and pushing them before the pilot could answer. Long story short, he is now Captain Gilad, a pilot.

Growing up in the air was fun. I learned to become a great sleeper and, by the age of five, I knew how much taxis should cost to JFK airport. I loved the thrill of waking up in the middle of the night to catch a plane, although I did enjoy the rare occasion of a nice relaxing trip, where we only had to (I should say, "got to") go to the airport once and then we could enjoy the rest of the trip. Okay, that was only once, but I will never forget the cruise to Alaska.

Later in life, after moving to Israel, we traveled a little less and I started to fear flying. The days of a fourteen-hour flight during which I slept the whole flight, even when the oxygen masks accidentally dropped, were done. I began the journey of staring at the map on the screen and I couldn't take my eyes off it, in fear that I would not have "control" of the plane anymore if I looked away. When there was turbulence, I would turn to a flight attendant and ask if they were scared. Thank God I'm overcoming those fears as we speak. (I'm on a plane right now, and I'm able to type this without staring at the screen — that counts as a major triumph!)

I used to get asked a lot what my hobbies were. I always responded that I didn't have any. Until I realized that traveling is a hobby. I got a thrill from traveling and it really helped my mental health, as well. In therapy, they suggest that you do things that make you happy as often as possible, to schedule events or plans that you can look forward to. You, Mommy, and my therapist asked if I'd like to have trips scheduled so that I'd have things to look forward to. And thank God for that!

Growing up, I thought that traveling was fun. Now I realize that traveling also has a purpose. For me, it's the best antidepressant out there. Maybe it's tied with Daisy and Buddy, my two dogs who have really helped me on my mental health journey.

Having a father in the travel business definitely had its ups and downs. The times you were away were really difficult and for me personally, it got harder as I got older. Working in the travel business means you're always working. Home or abroad. It also exhausted you so much that sometimes, on the rare occasion when you didn't have to work, you were so tired you couldn't commit to doing things with us.

When you had that pulmonary embolism, we realized how harmful traveling could be. Thank God (and thank Ilan and Gilad) you got to the hospital right on time and were saved.

On the other hand, your traveling has resulted in saving many lives. Helping Syrian refugees, attending the aftermath of hurricanes, floods, earthquakes, and other natural disasters. You've helped countless others, strangers, but you've also traveled to help me, flying me around the US to get help with my mental health.

You attended tons of conferences of all different kinds. You spread Zionism everywhere you went (well, at least we convinced you not to try in Syria). You spread the importance of mental health everywhere. Those good deeds wouldn't have been possible without travel.

One trip I remember as life-changing was with Masa Hashemesh, that "sunlight journey" group. You organized a trip in 2012 for me and some other kids my age, a group of Israeli teens volunteering to go to New York state and help rebuild after the destruction caused by Hurricane Sandy. We also rallied for the support of Israel in general, through *hasbara,* a term that means "advocacy" or "explanation."

People are always so amazed by all the good deeds you do and the help you offer. I feel bad about not being as appreciative as others of the things you do, but I was spoiled by you and Mommy always doing these amazing things so that nothing ever surprised me. I took your good deeds for granted.

We've lived in several places, but "lived" is a very hard to define word. I see it that I had the opportunity to live in many places and the misfortune to do so, as well. You've been known in myriad ways at various places; stops along life's path. When you arrive at hotels where you frequently stay, they'll greet you warmly as "Mr. Katz." You've been known as President (of the synagogue). Saba Stu (grandpa in Hebrew) and Abba (father in Hebrew). Mr. Kate's (some foreign clients who had trouble pronouncing your name). The One Who Is Always Pacing (as you are a Fitbit addict never wanting to scrimp on steps). The One Who Won't Take No for an Answer (you've been known to be stubborn ... on occasion). The Israeli, the American, the Panamanian (depending on which passport you use). The traveler, the travel agent. The One Who Won't Forgo Even One Ounce in a Suitcase (you take seriously your allotment of three suitcases at seventy pounds each when you fly, even throwing in a box of cereal or roll of toilet paper to make sure each suitcase gives me full value at 69.9 pounds of content). While the Sabalim (porters in Hebrew) know you as Stuart, in Hebrew סטוארט. Maybe one day you'll be known as Dr. Stuart Katz. I will always feel the joy of hearing my favorite name of mine: "Wow, are you Stuart and Carol Katz's daughter?"

I have stayed at places where you literally traveled thousands of miles just to be able to visit me through a window in the freezing cold. You have walked miles in the snow to be able to visit me on Shabbat. Although that time you fell in a ditch while I was going to shul ... I'm not responsible for that one.

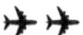

In listening to my children's recollections, I'm struck with several thoughts that may provide insight to other parents considering how to travel with their families. One is linked just to my family, but to read that each of my children would choose Australia if they could go anywhere in the world means that future Katz family journeys should be on my to-do list, although it'll be tough to coordinate with all of our crazy schedules.

We parents think we know what's happening with our kids, and then they'll surprise us. When Ilan told me that he most enjoyed cruises growing up, I was thrown for a loop. Carol and I will never forget Ilan's comment when we were on the Alaska Cruise and were going through some glaciers. We called him to come to our balcony to witness some of the most incredible sites he would ever see. His reply: "If this is going to be the most incredible thing I see, my life is really bad ...." This bummed us out at the time — what can a parent do, other than bring their kid to something they think is memorable, wonderful, and see what happens? But it turns out that the cruises were a hit. Who knew?

People — kids especially — remember surprises and firsts better than anything else. Books on the art of memory, *ars memoriae*, note this as well. If every day you paraglide, then paragliding becomes quotidian and no longer noteworthy. If you go only once, then the experience is forever etched in your memory. If you walk the same path to school each day, no matter how picturesque it is, then the memory merges into a single positive one, even if those walks took place over many years. But that one time that a watermelon fell from an upstairs apartment window and nearly clocked you in the head? You'll remember that one. One year we went on a family trip that didn't involve logically connected destinations, just those linked by a theme: canals. We visited Amsterdam, London, Venice, and Panama. We lived in New York at the time, so you don't need to be a geography guru or travel agent to realize this makes no sense logistically, but that was part of the appeal. It was a surrealist trip. Gilad and I loved it. The others were along for the ride. Literally, riding each canal we visited. Sometimes weird works just because it's weird, and therefore memorable, a talking point.

With this in mind, we parents can curate surprises, distinctive moments, firsts, building them into travel plans. My family did this with entire trips, playing The Game in which we wouldn't tell our kids where we were going, or not all the details, letting them try to guess, or pulling a fast one and letting them think we're going one place when the final destination was elsewhere. They enjoyed it at the time and it's reassuring to learn that now, as adults, that game remains a happy memory.

But nothing is black and white. Dafna loved almost all our time playing "The Game," until that time when she didn't.

We'd been in Baltimore for a family reunion and were headed out on one of our surprise trips. Carol's grandmother had just died, and this felt like a good time to get away, after a tough period. We flew from Baltimore to Dallas then to Tokyo. The kids thought we were at our destination, but Carol and I had thought what fun it would be to pull a fast one. To be fair, it had been considered great fun on past trips. But when we passed out Hong Kong dollars to the kids, revealing that Tokyo was not, in fact, the final destination, Dafna burst into tears. She was at a point where the idea of yet another flight, even a shortish one (around four hours) from Tokyo to Hong Kong, was more than she could deal with.

Parents often respond with dismay about how few specifics of their children's youthful moments of discovery and happiness their kids actually remember. For parents, they are glowing memories, like embers in the sand. For the kids, they are pieces in a vast mosaic called childhood that is about the feeling produced by the mosaic, not really about the individual pieces of it. Kids remember their childhood, or eras within it, as happy or stressful, difficult, or prosperous. Some of the mosaic tiles will stand out — individual moments, usually of extreme emotion (joy, sadness) or surprise (expecting two cars but getting a limo loaded with Diet Coke). But they gloss over the details. A primary goal from us parents is to create a safe, consistently positive, and supportive environment — a happy mosaic. It can be full of particularly beautiful individual tiles, but we can't expect the kids to remember them as we do. Success is when our kids look back on their childhoods as overall blanketed in lack of want and scattered with moments of true joy.

* The canal-themed holiday was London, Amsterdam, Venice, and Panama (we tried to get Cairo in there, to do the Suez Canal, but the dates and flights didn't work out.)

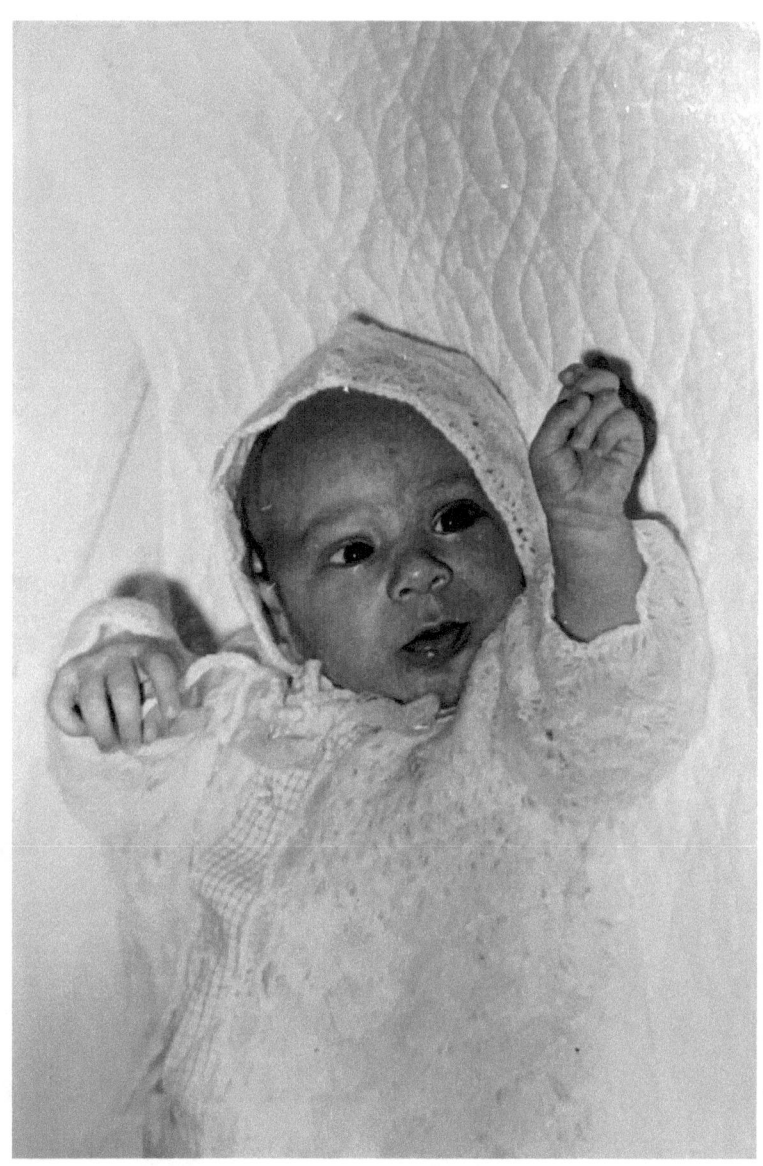

Stuart, one month old.

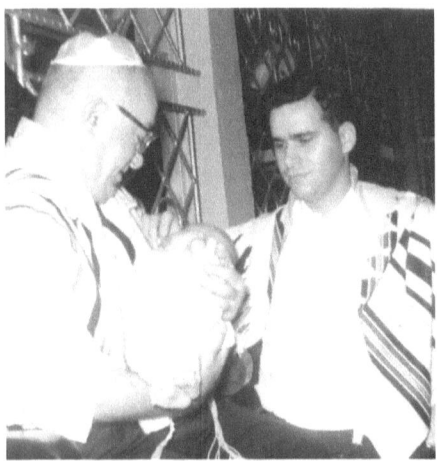
Stuart's Brit Milah, with his father and Zaddie Katz (foreskin not pictured).

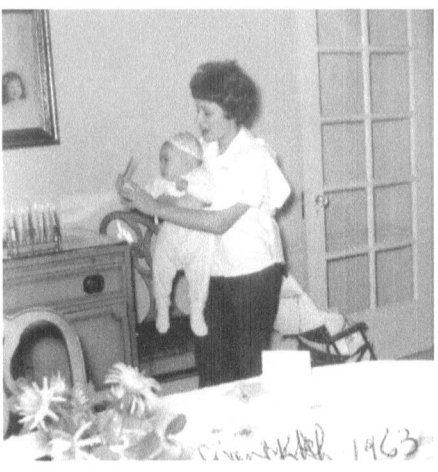
Stuart's first Chanukah.

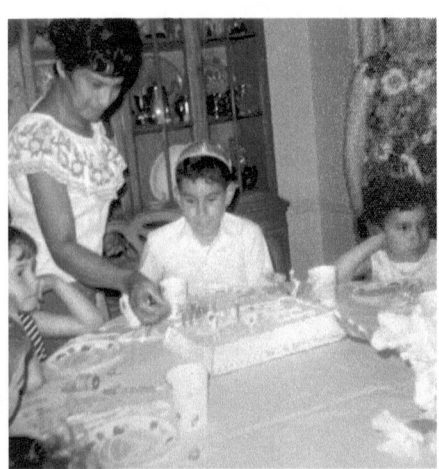
Apparently, Stuart did have birthday parties. Shown here with siblings and Mima.

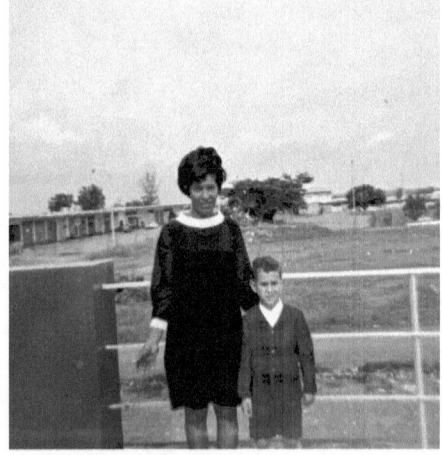
Beloved nanny Mima and young Stuart.

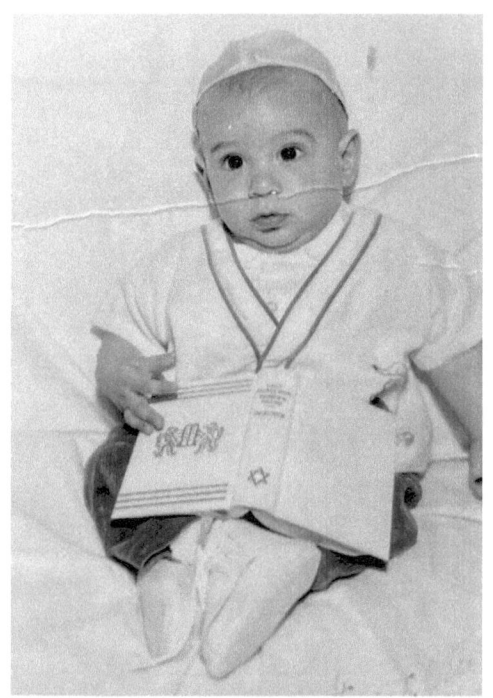

Stuart's first Siddur.

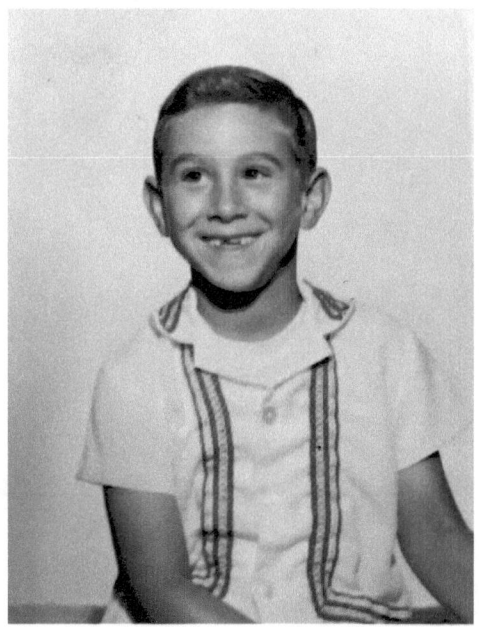

Age six.

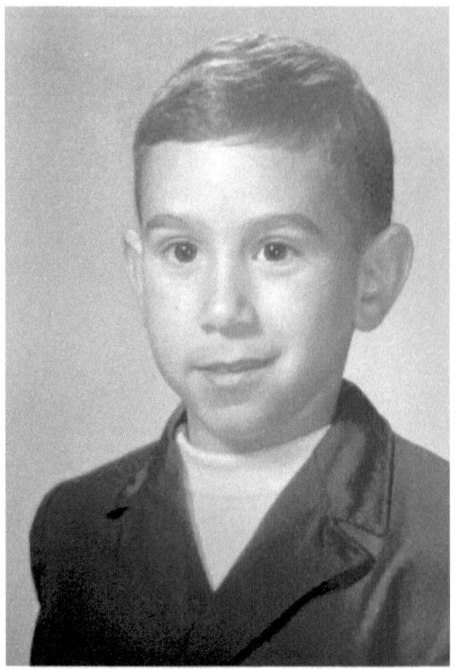

Age seven.

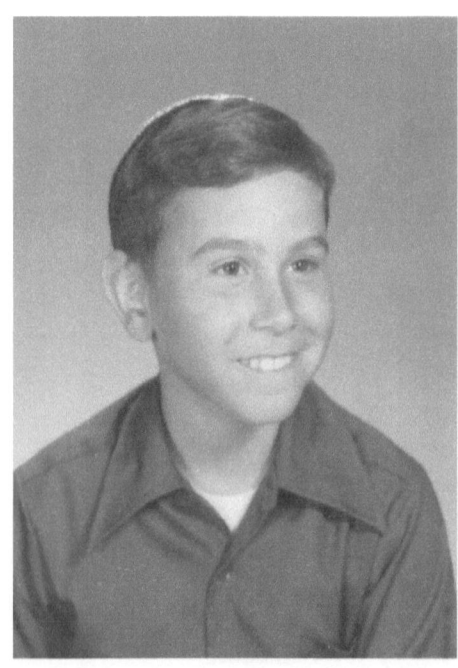

Age nine.

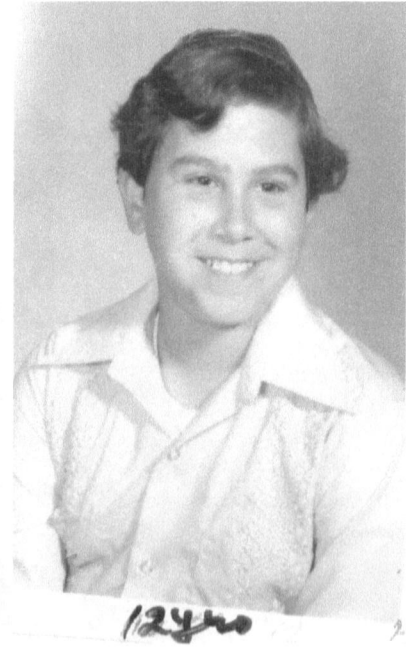

Age twelve.

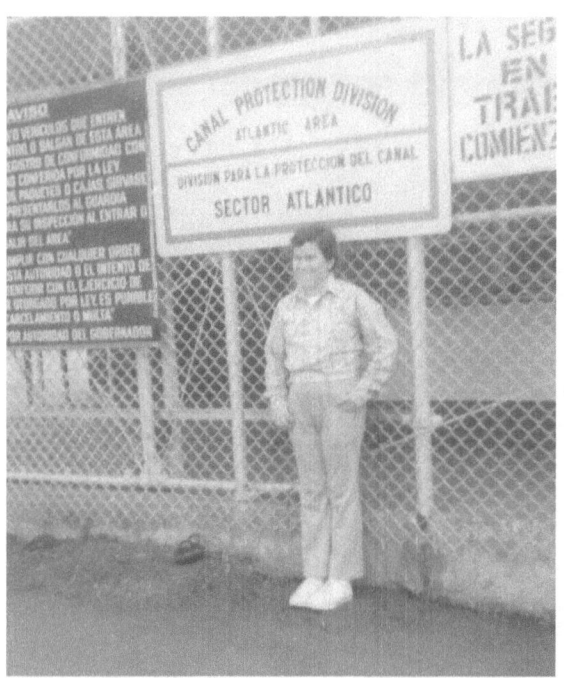

Stuart at the Panama Canal.

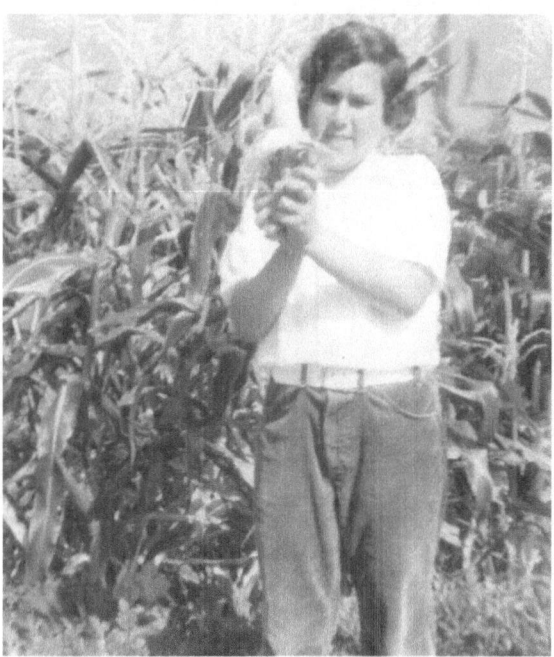

Stuart, aged twelve, in his backyard corn field.

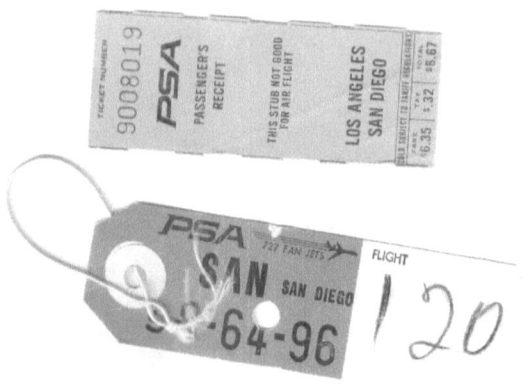

Bag tag and ticket from Stuart's first solo flight—age four.

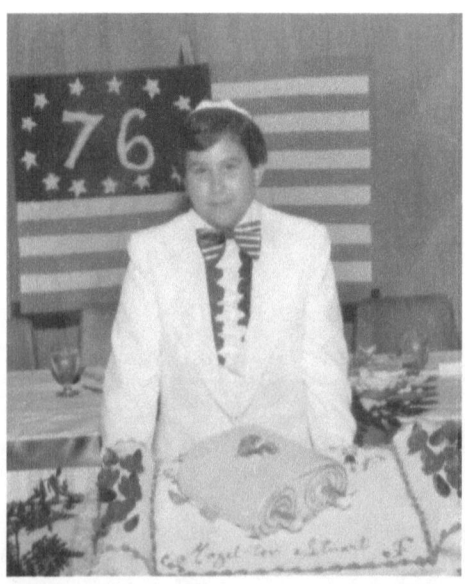

Stuart's Bar Mitzvah, featuring torah-shaped cake!

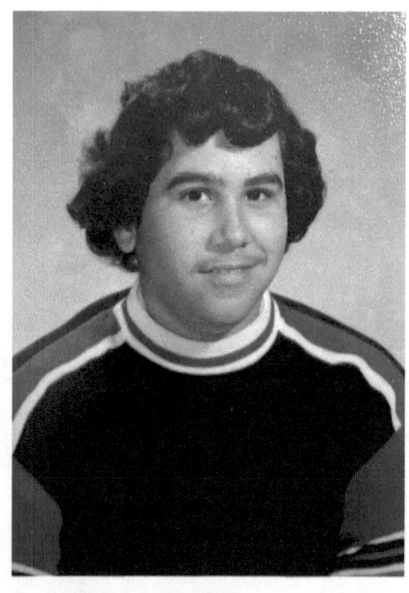

Stuart's awkward years.

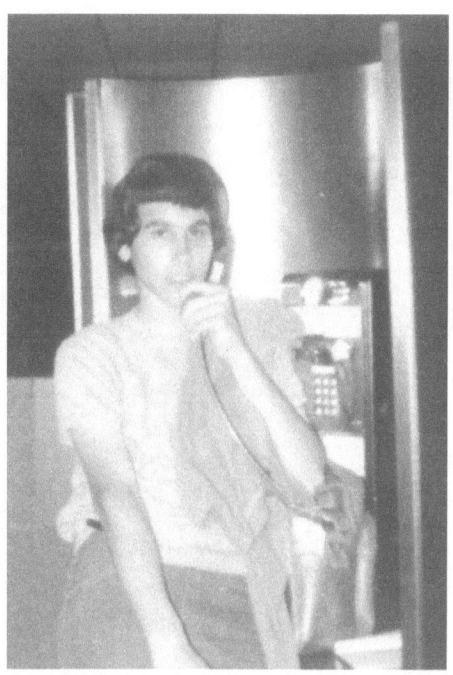

Stuart on a payphone, his only means of communication while at boarding school.

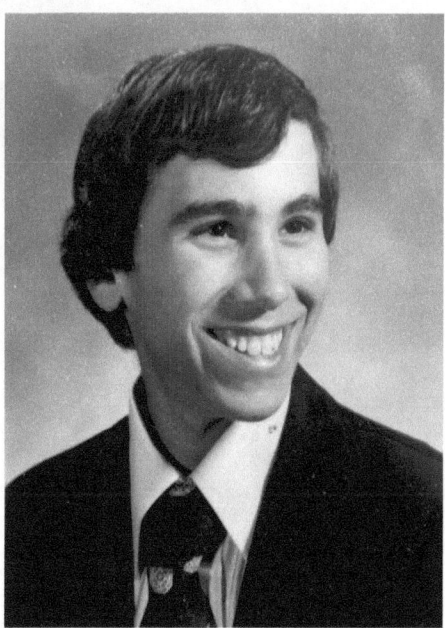

A high school yearbook photo.

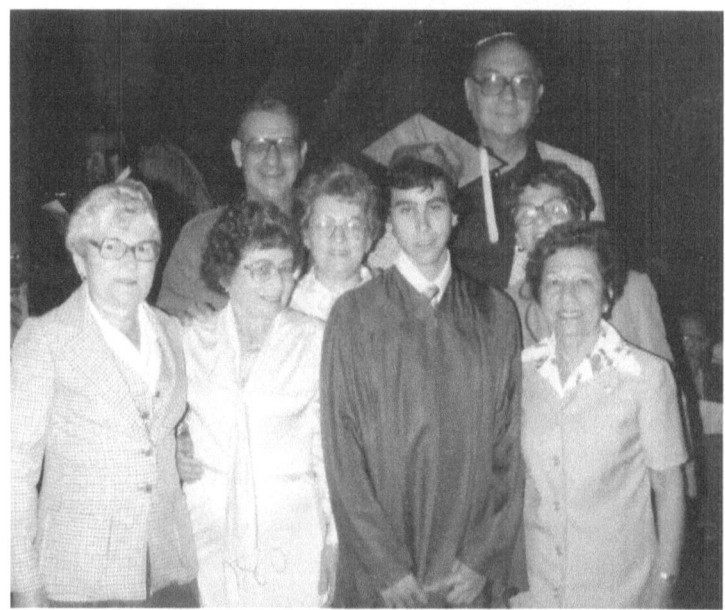

High School graduation with the family in tow.

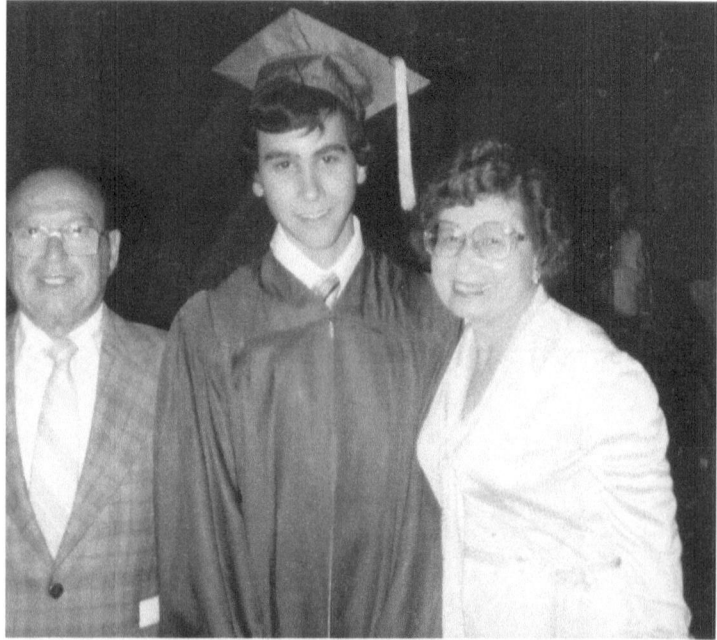

High School graduation, flanked by Bubbie and Zaddie Andelman.

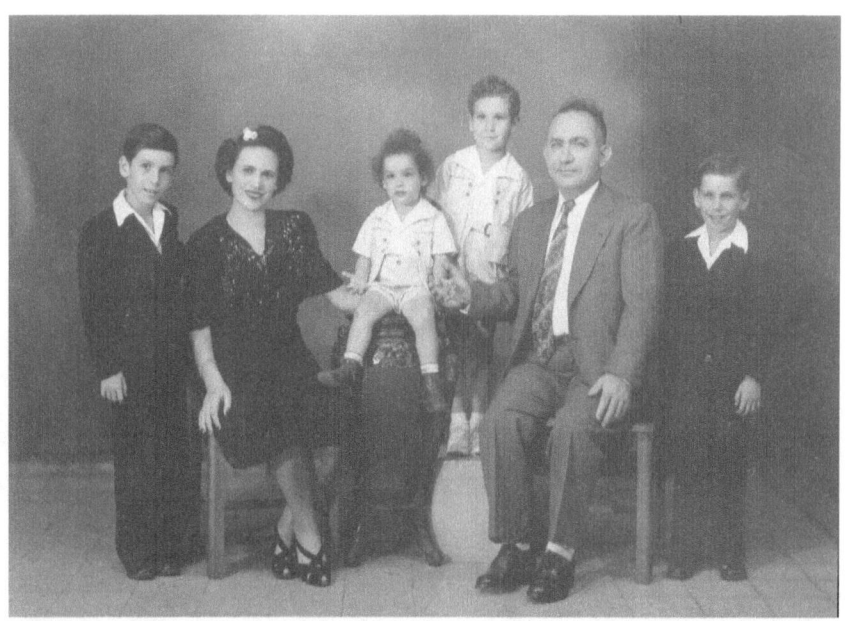

Bubbie and Zaddie Katz with their four boys.

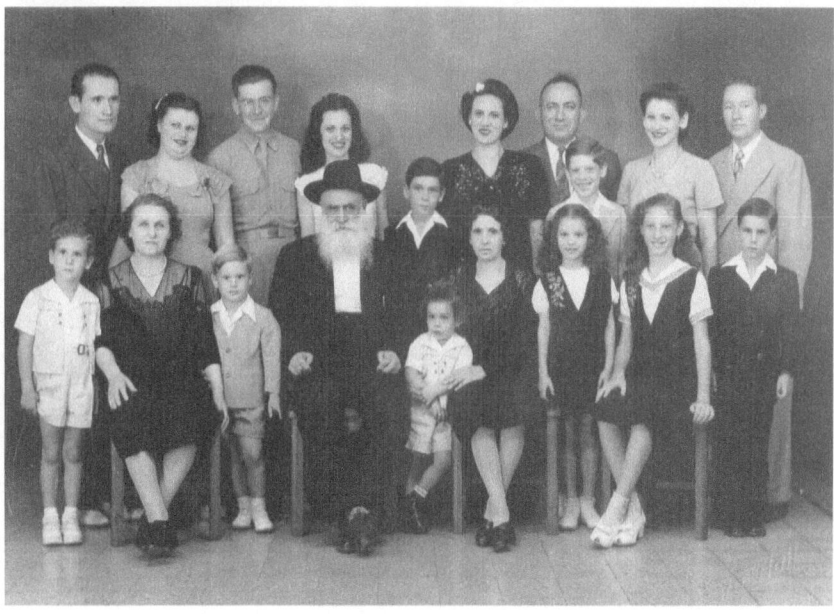

The Eisen family (Bubbie Katz's relatives), photographed in 1946 in Colon, Panama.

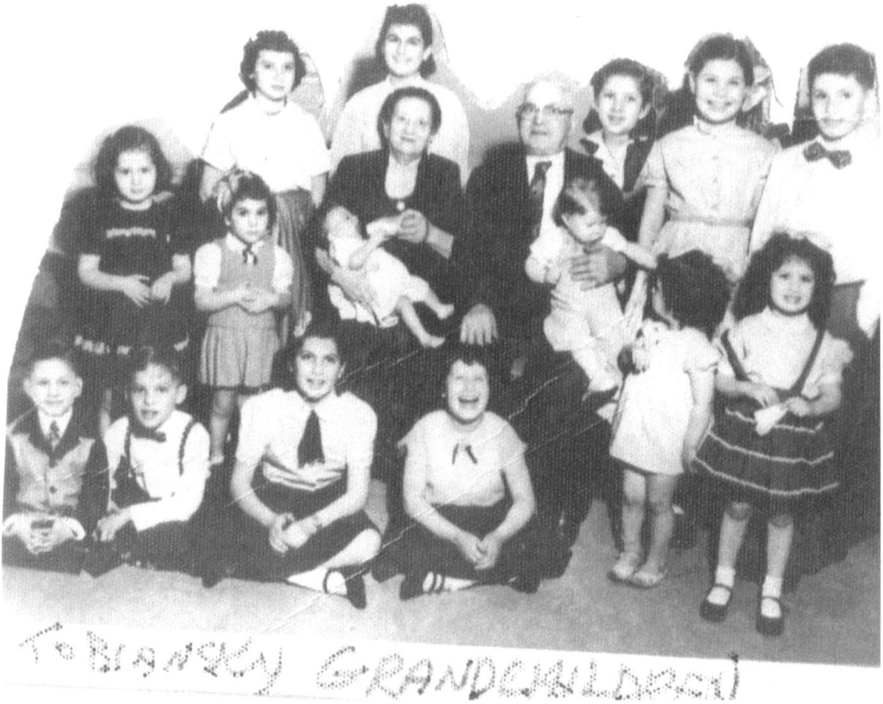

Bubbie Andelman's family, the Tobiansky grandchildren.

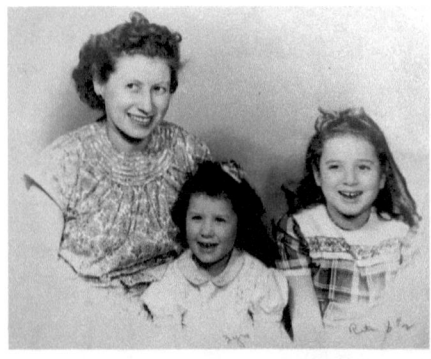

Young Bubbie Andelman with her daughters: Stuart's mom and Aunt Elayne.

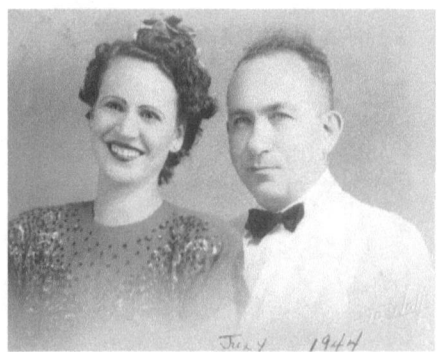

Bubbie and Zaddie Katz looking sharp.

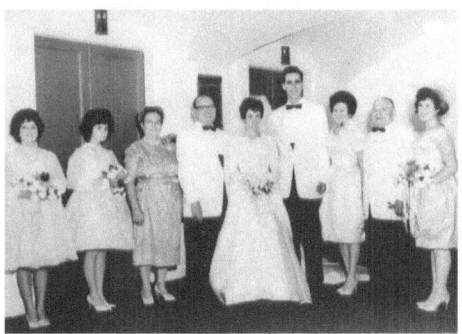
The wedding of Stuart's parents.

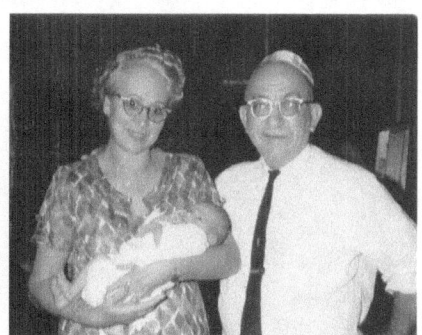
Bubbie and Zaddie Katz holding newborn Stuart.

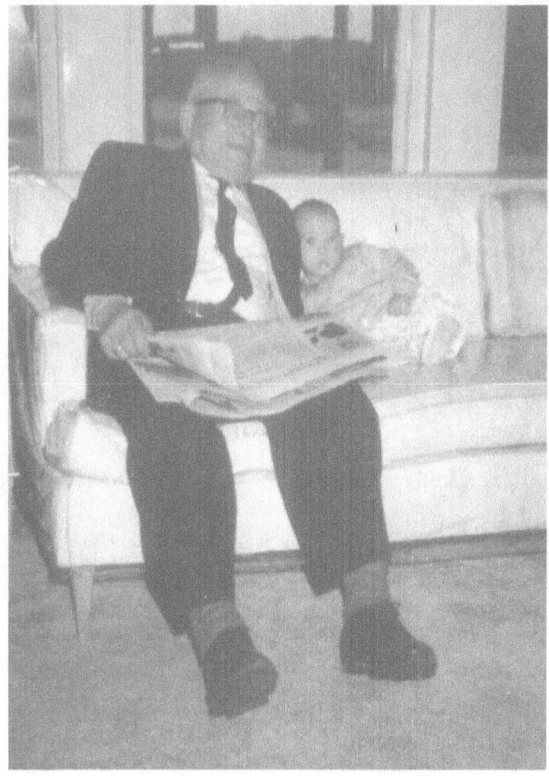
"Papa" Zaddie Tobiansky reading all the news that's fit to print with Stuart's help.

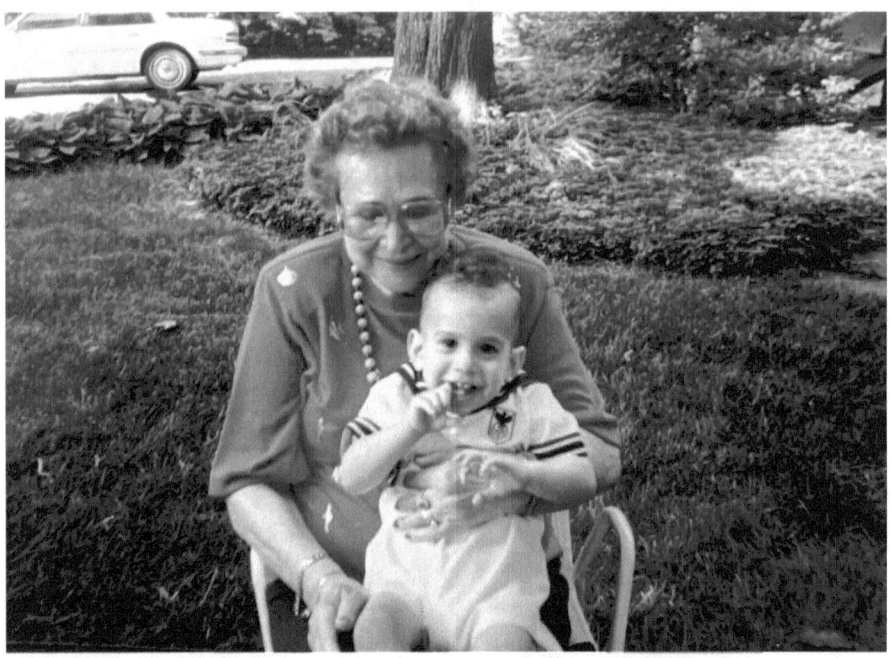

Bubbie Katz with baby Ilan.

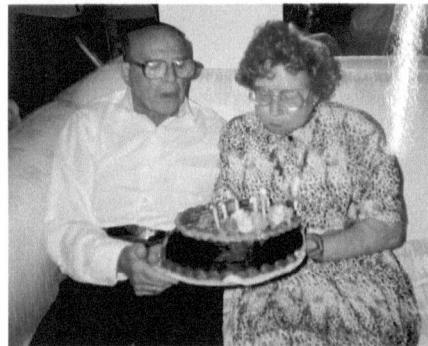

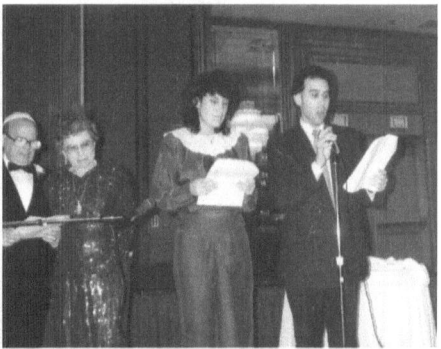

Bubbie and Zaddie Andelman had a longstanding bit that they'd do. Bubbie would say, "Shall we share a piece of cake." Zaddie would reply, "Yes, and I'll have one, too." Vaudeville here they come!

Stuart with his cousin Ethel at Bubbie and Zaddie Andelman's 50th wedding anniversary.

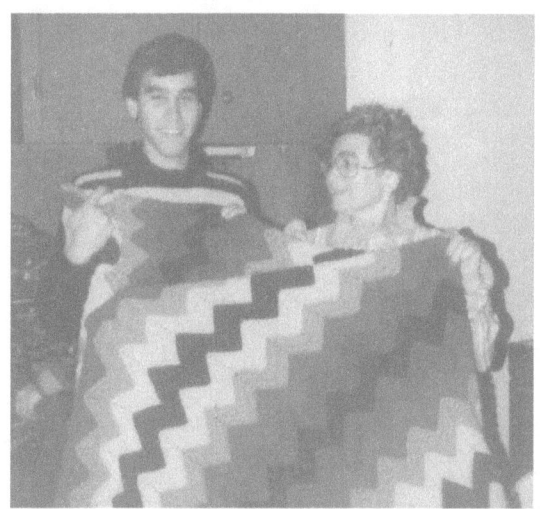

Bubbie Andelman knit a handmade blanket for each grandchild—this is Stuart's.

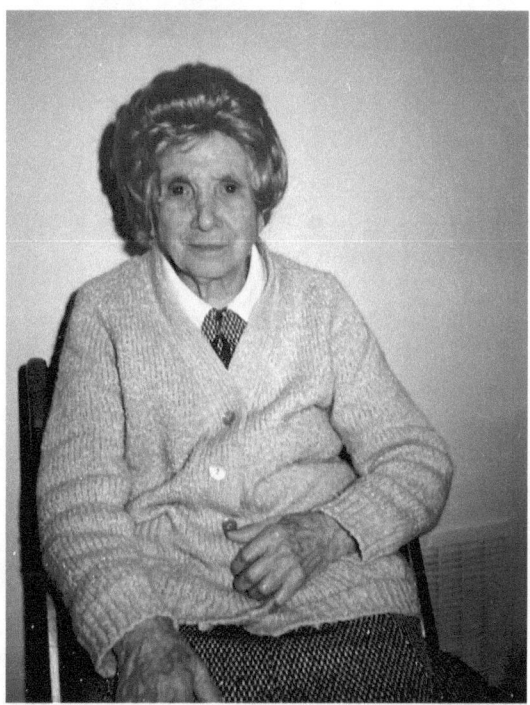

Bubbie Eisen.

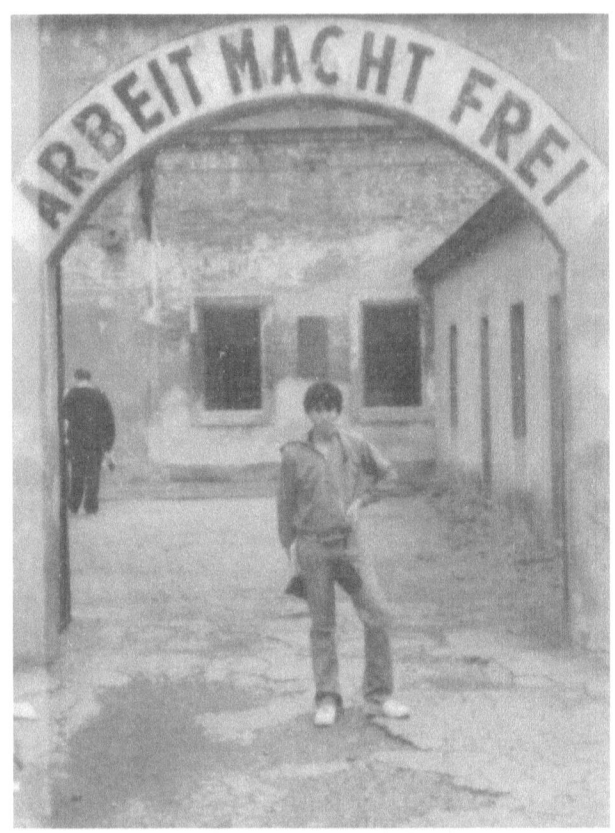

Visiting a concentration camp with the trick moto over the gate, "Works makes freedom."

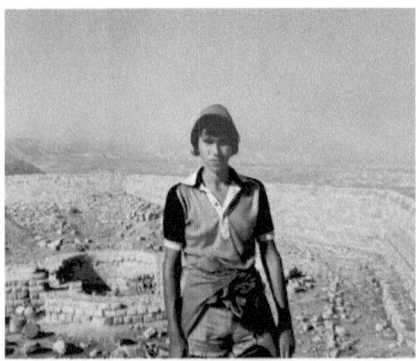

Walking in the Land of Israel, overlooking the Negev Desert.

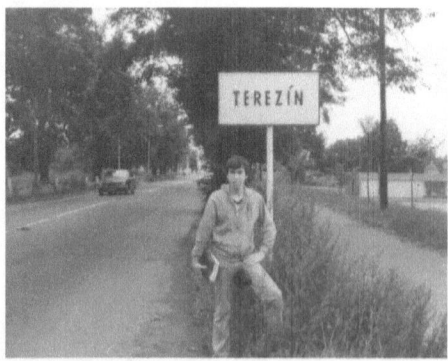

Abroad in Terezin, Czechoslovakia.

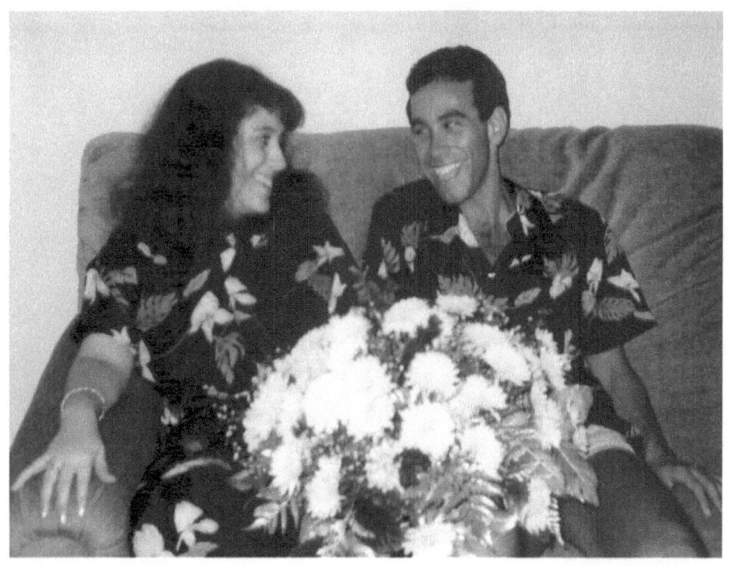

Carol and Stuart sharing a moment in celebration of their engagement.

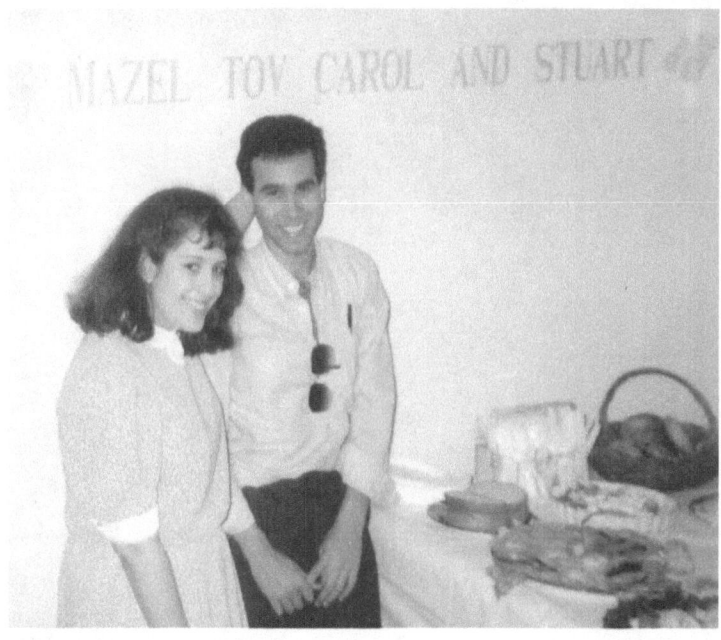

Everything always revolves around food, especially at the engagement party.

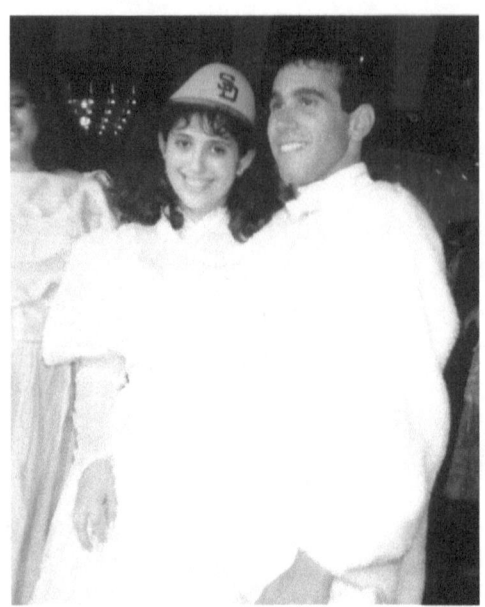

At their wedding, Stuart surprised Carol with a dance dressed as a bunny.

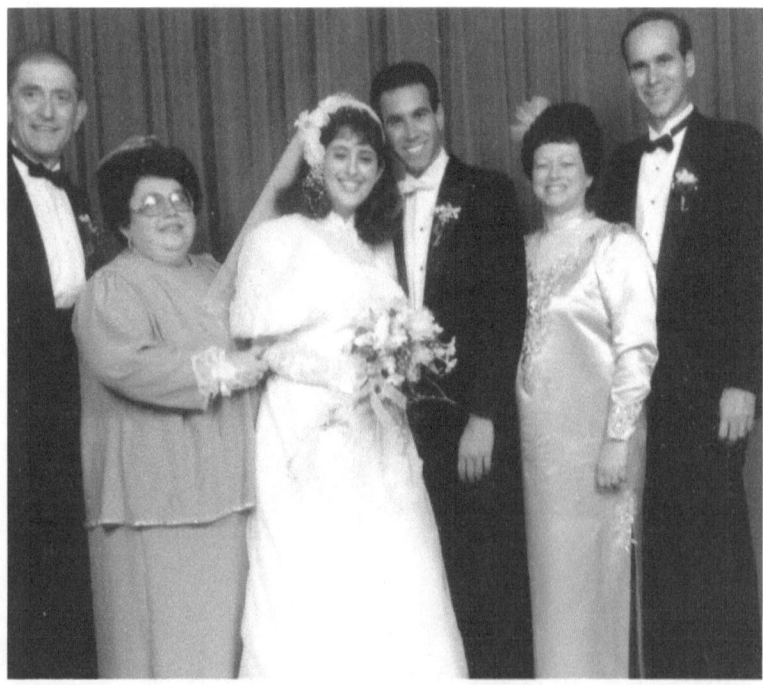

The bride and groom flanked by their parents.

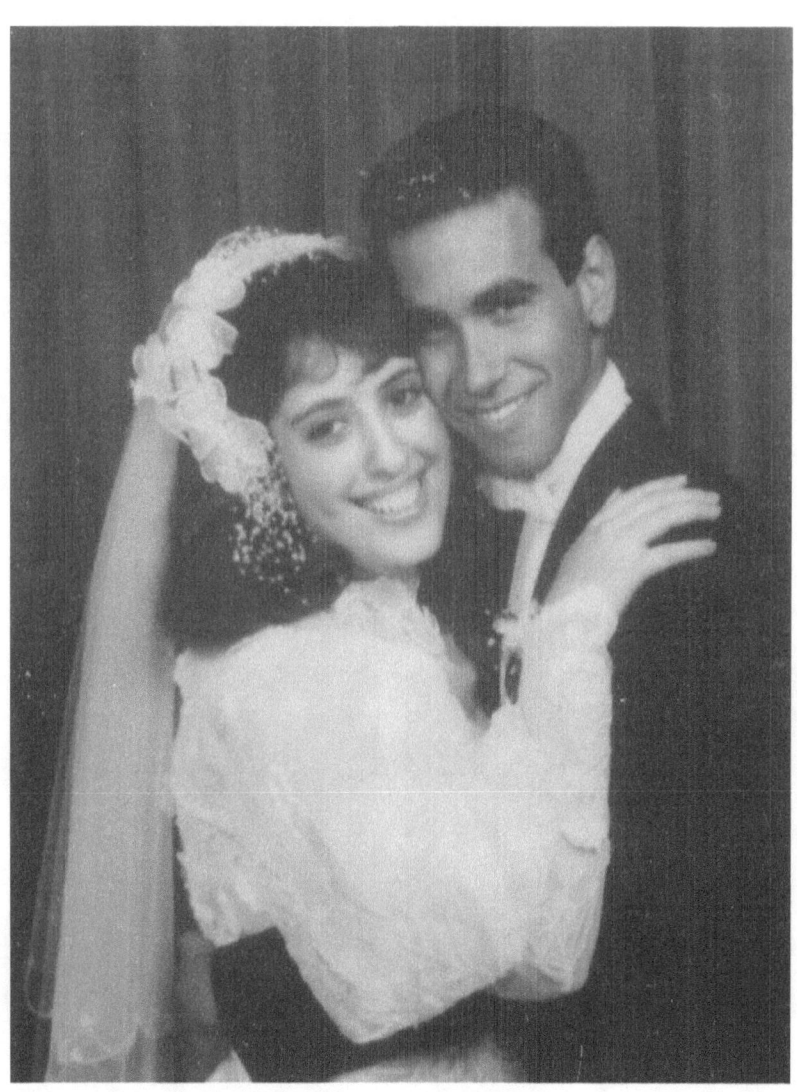

Stuart and Carol's wedding.

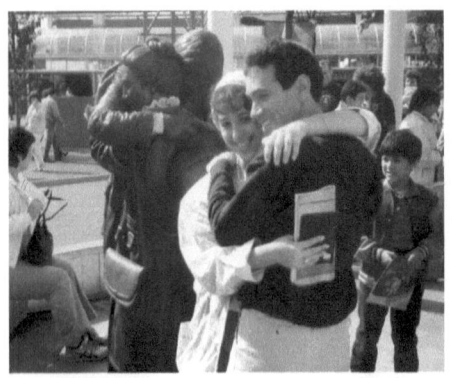

At the start of the honeymoon, prior to engaging in international espionage, here shown in Vancouver.

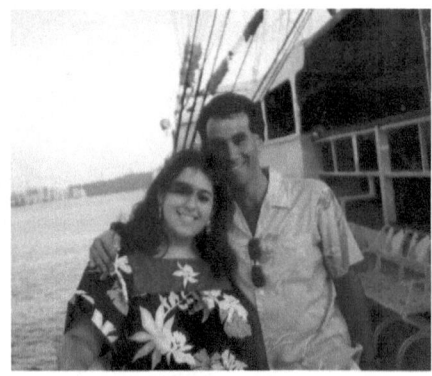

In Hawaii, the most-frequently-visited holiday spot (thank you Frequent Flyer Miles).

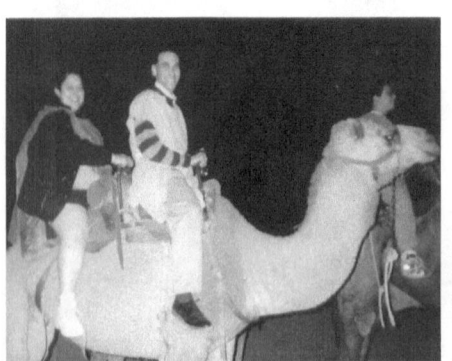

Riding a camel across the desert.

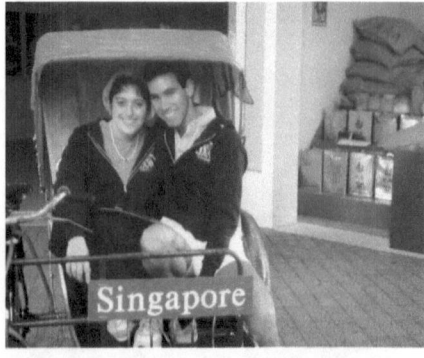

Rickshaw snuggles in Singapore.

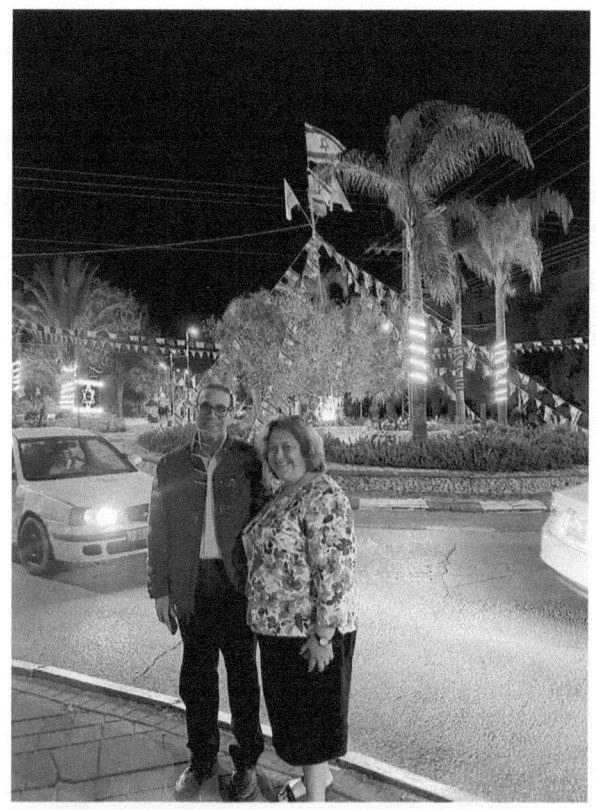

In Hashmonaim on Israel Independence Day.

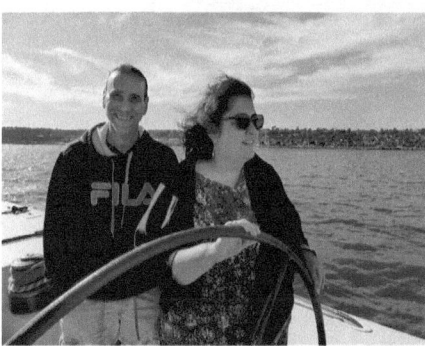

Sailing aboard America's Cup.

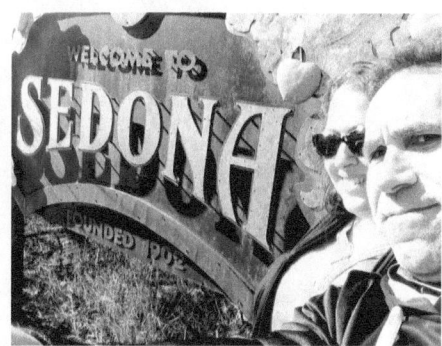

In Sedona, Arizona.

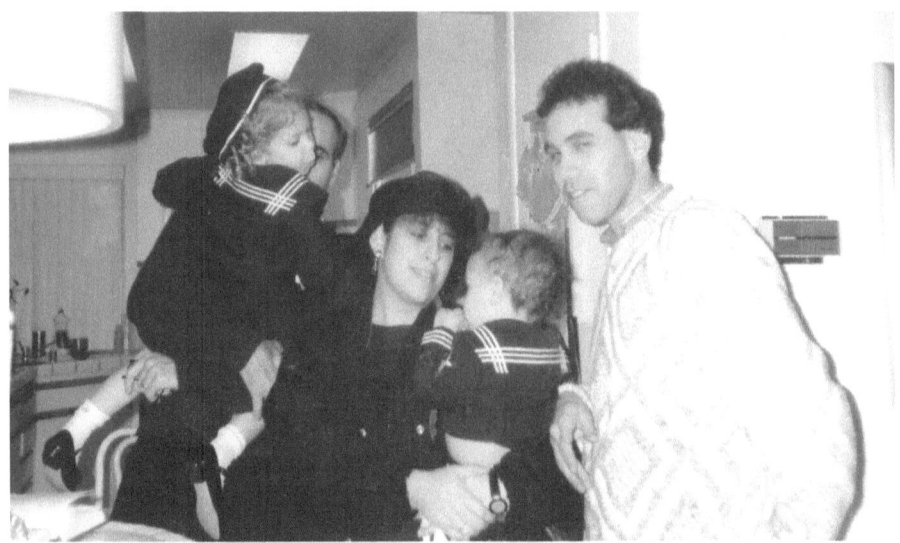

Carol and Stuart balancing Adina and Ilan.

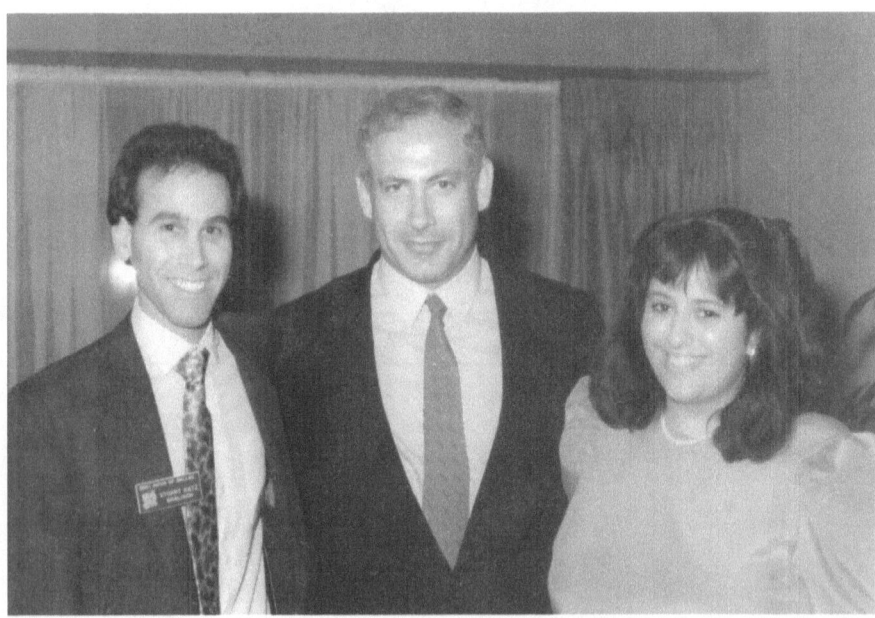

In the company of Benjamin Netanyahu at a Bnei Akiva dinner in Dallas.

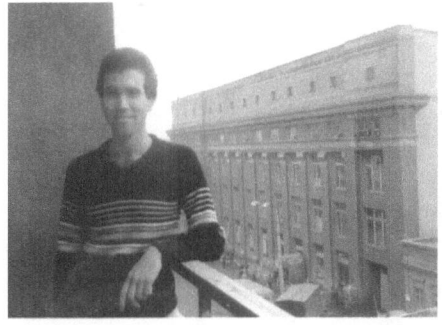

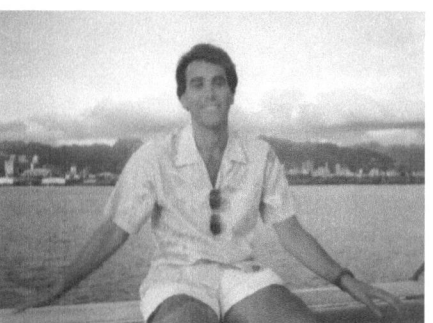

Stuart in his secret agent days, posing in the Soviet Union.

In Hawaii—always a favorite destination.

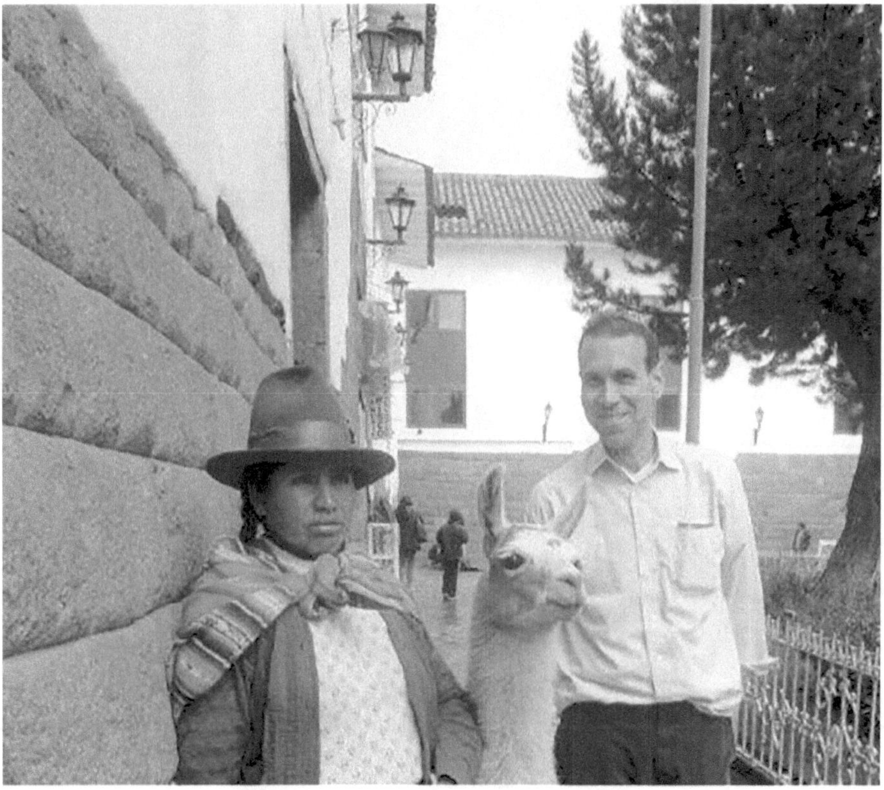

In Cuzco, Peru.

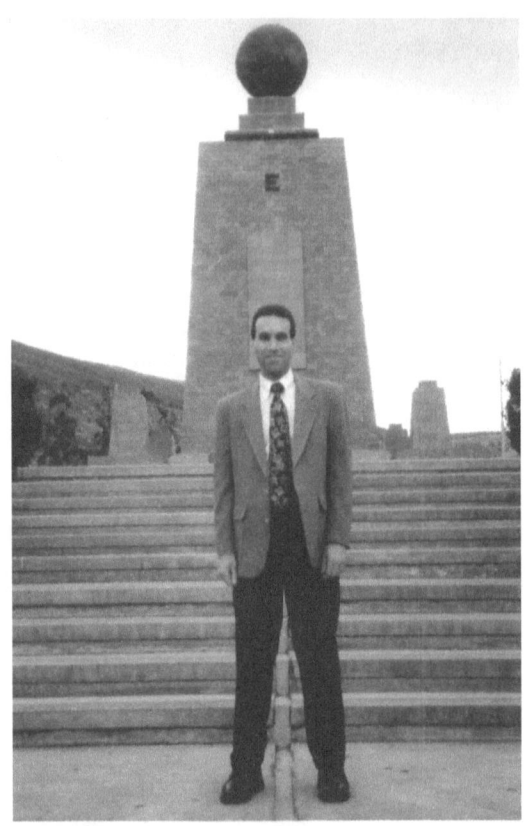

Straddling the equator in Ecuador.

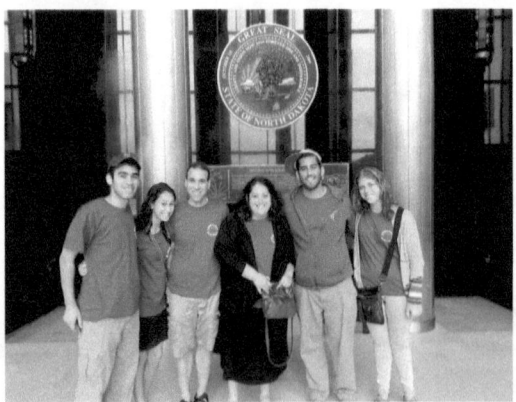

On a family trip to Stuart's 50th US state—the one and only North Dakota.

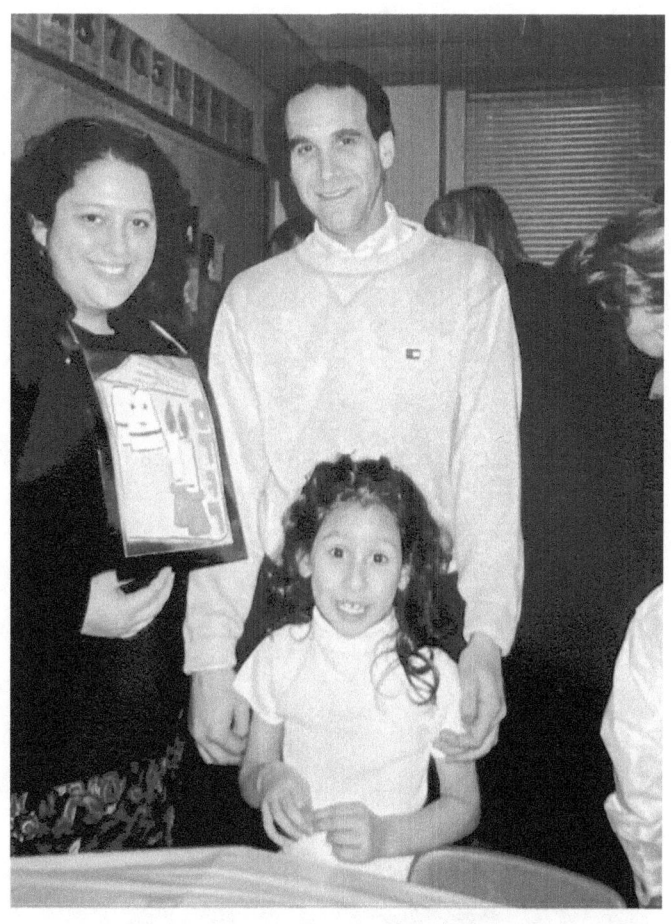

Stuart and Carol at Dafna's Siddur party.

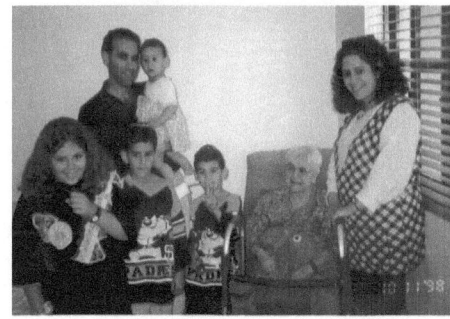

Stuart, Carol and Kids.

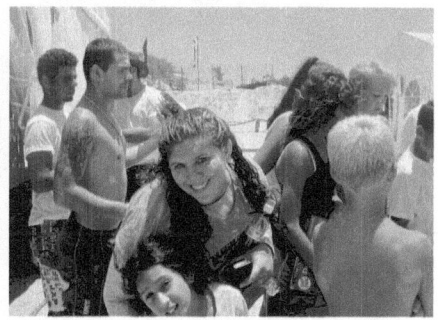

Adina and Dafna helping displaced people in 2006.

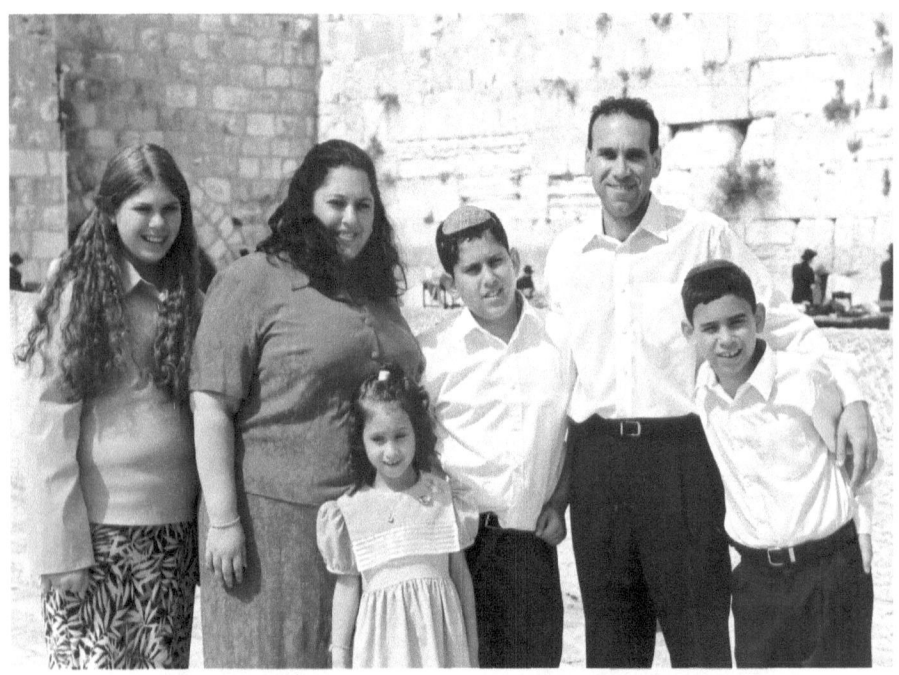

Posing in front of Jerusalem's Western Wall at Ilan's Bar Mitzah.

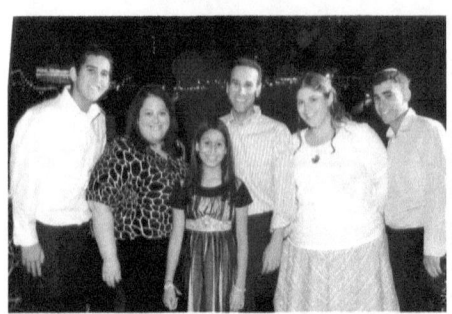

The kids and Carol at Dafna's Bat Mitzvah.

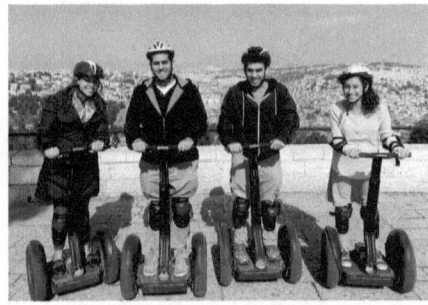

The kids on Segways in Jerusalem.

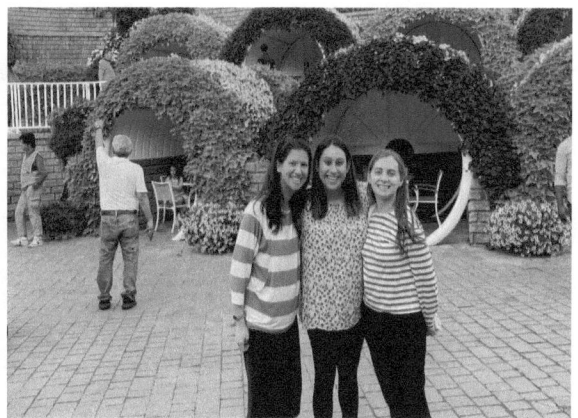

Dafna, Margalit and Naomi in Dubai.

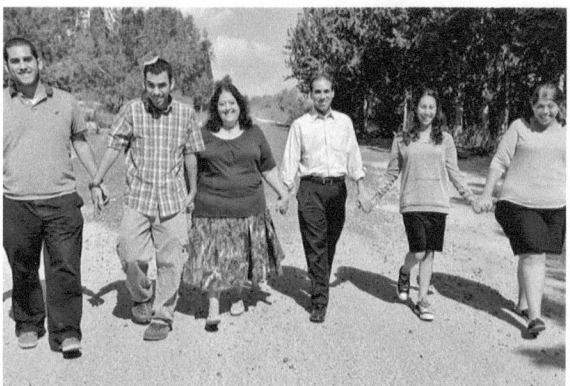

The Katz Six.

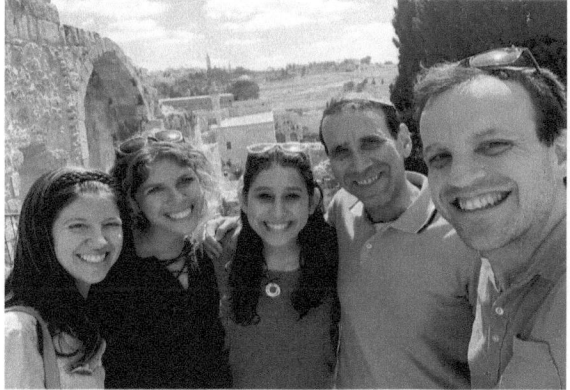

In the hills of Jerusalem, with Ophir, Adina, Margalit and Dafna.

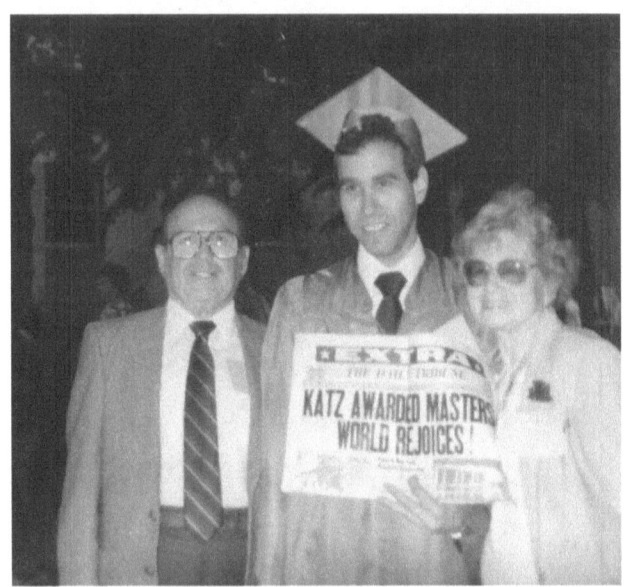

Grad school graduation at Columbia, which made headlines, alongside Bubbie and Zaddie Andelman.

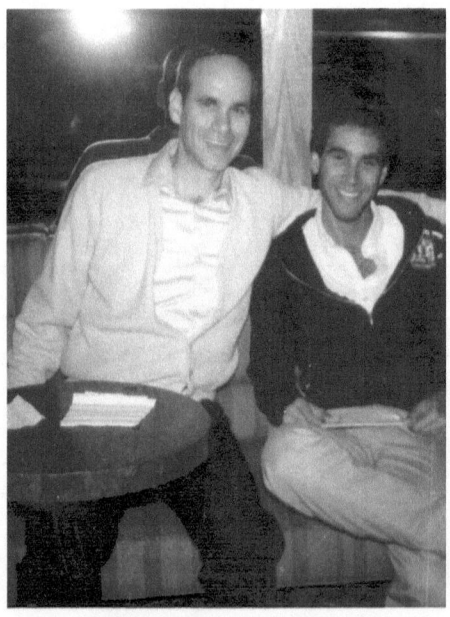

Stuart with his father.

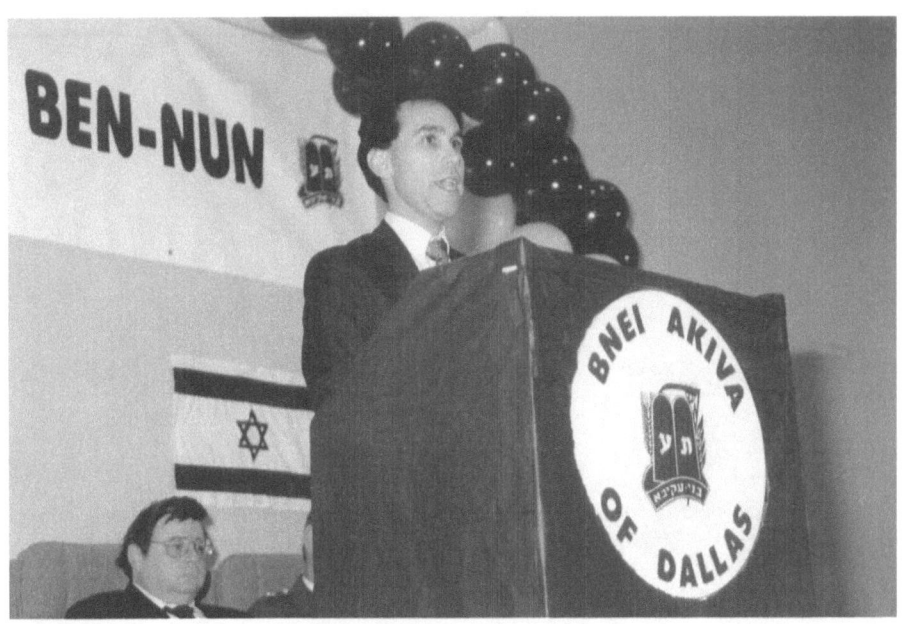
Speaking at an event for the Dallas branch of Bnei Akiva.

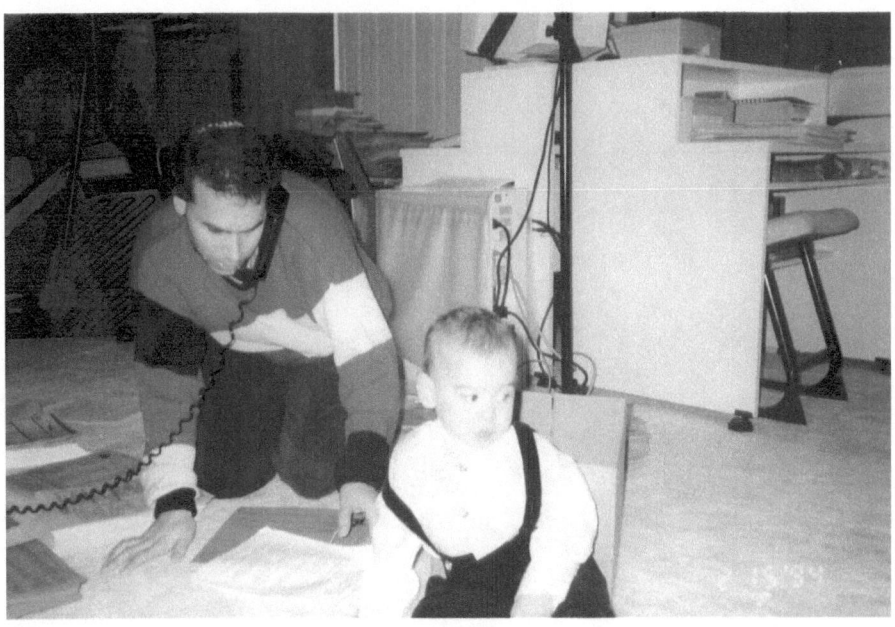
Stuart multitasking as usual, with baby Gilad lending a hand.

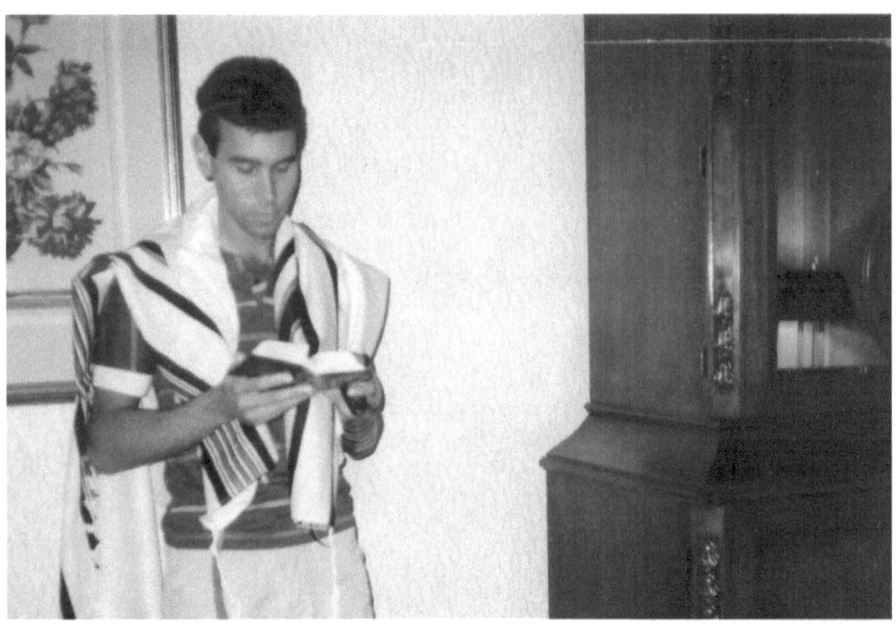

In prayer.

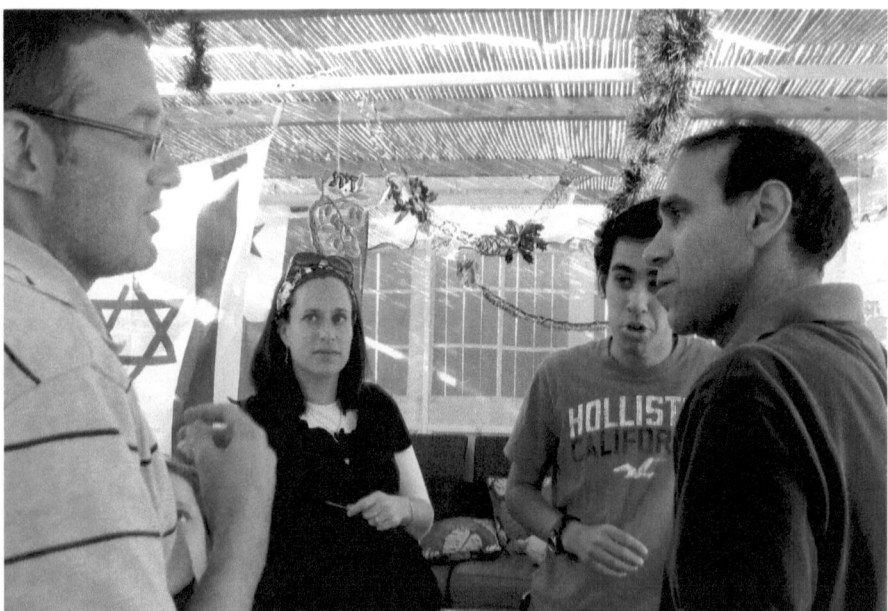

An Andelman family gathering for Sukkot, with cousins David and Shira, alongside Gilad and Stuart.

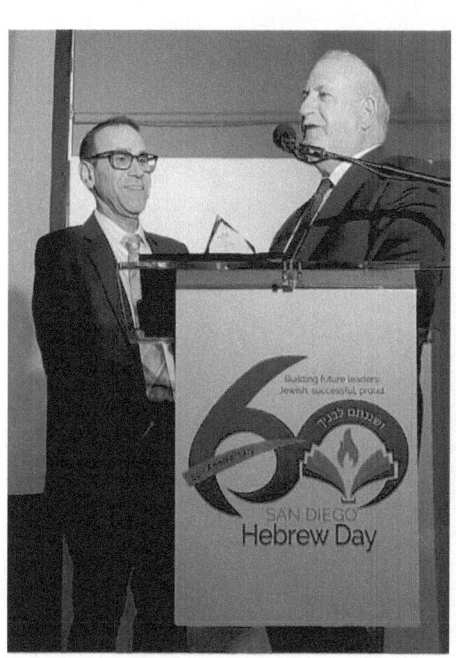 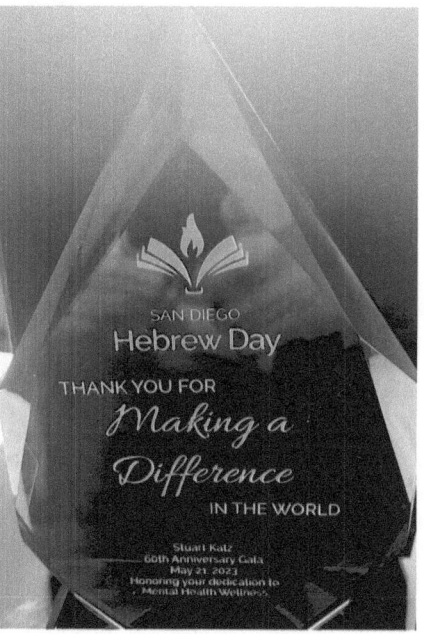

Recognized as Alumnus of the Year at San Diego Hebrew Day School—on the day that both the school and Stuart turned sixty.

The award presented by Rabbi Weiser.

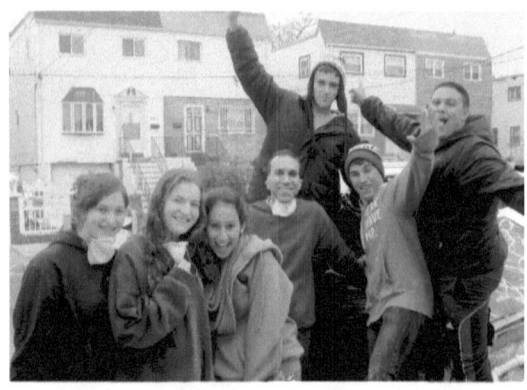

Our team during the Masa Hashemesh volunteer trip on Long Island.

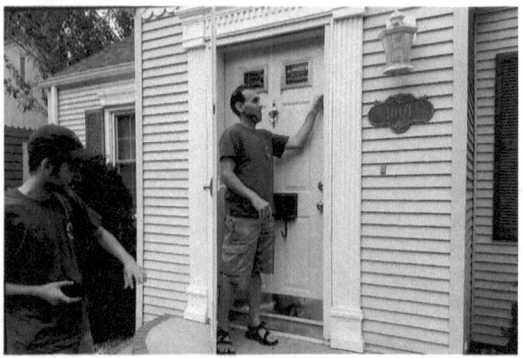

Adding the finishing touch by hanging a mezuzah on the doorpost in North Dakota.

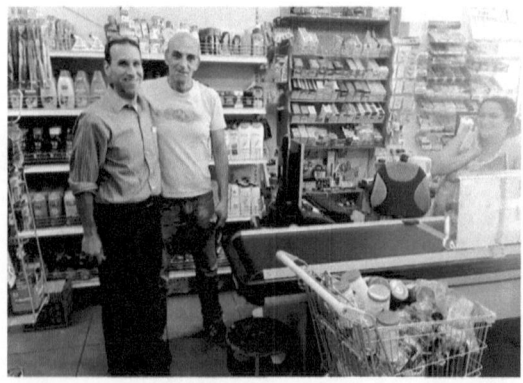

Stuart and Ilan Chen at a market in Sderot, buying groceries for a family in need.

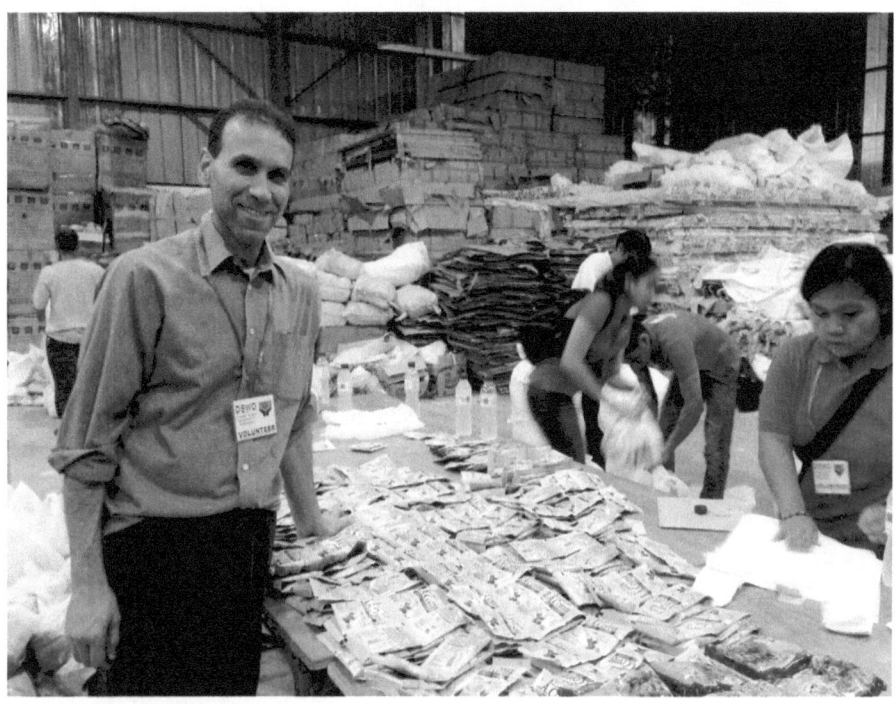

Helping pack emergency supplies in Manila.

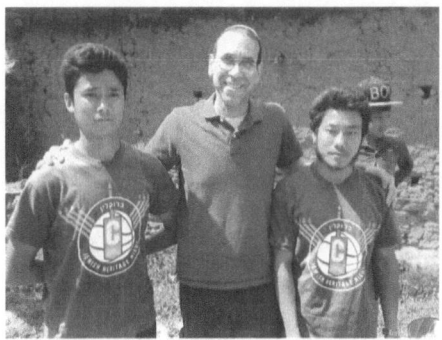

Stuart in a Nepali rice field as part of his volunteer work. Somehow these two locals had on Jewish Heritage Night t-shirts!

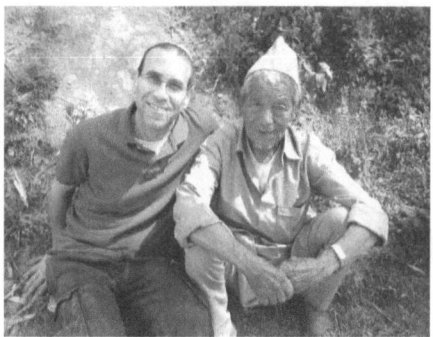

Stuart with a victim of the earthquake in Nepal.

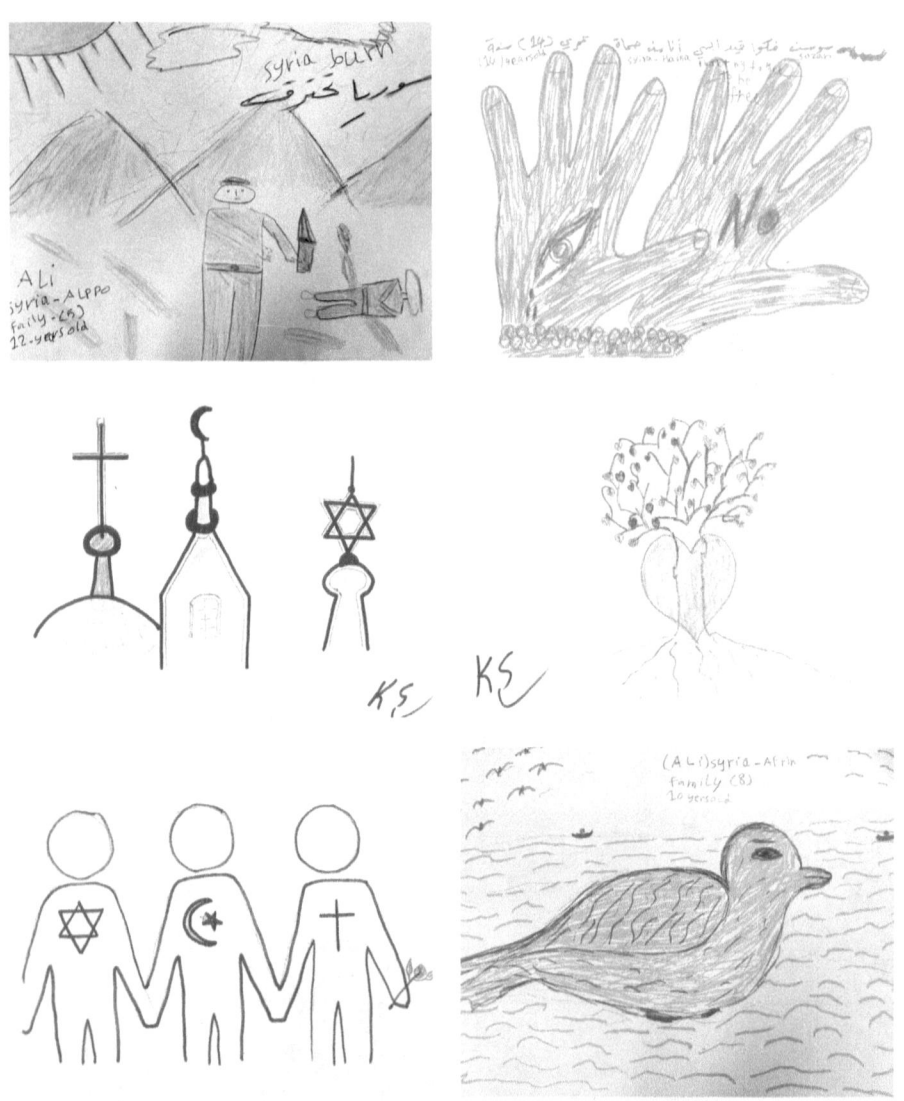

Drawings by refugee children, gifted to Stuart in thanks for his help.

Chapter 12

Travel for Volunteer Work

Philippines

No society can understand itself without looking at its shadow side.

— Gabor Maté

Whatever issues may have worked their way into my own family, they pale in comparison to the plight of those suffering in the wake of immediate, catastrophic events, like war, famine, and weather-related disasters. Hearing of such tragedies in the news brings out another side of my paternal instinct — I want to help.

In 2013, the news was filled with accounts of the devastation in the Philippines following a typhoon. More than two million were displaced, thousands killed, tens of thousands injured. The economy was likewise devastated.

By this point it will come as no surprise that I set off as soon as I could, to offer what help I could. But this trip would prove to be a special one, for there I found a true love for Jews in a country of Catholics, a love that I did not anticipate.

I landed in Manila, planning to get started volunteering first thing the next morning. However, while on the tarmac and witnessing numerous C-130 military aircraft with what seemed to be evacuees disembarking, I was seized with the feeling that I should rush to help, jet lag and settling in be damned. My taxi driver was fascinated to learn that I'd come from Israel. He was effusive in his praise for the Jewish People. I kept wondering, "Is he serious or just after a big tip?" but he sounded so sincere I truly believed him.

He also told me that if I really wanted to help, I should go to Tacloban. He took me to a friend of his and set me up to go to Tacloban on Thursday, but that was two days away — I wanted to help now.

After checking in at the hotel and making some calls, I headed out to the Civil Aviation Authority of the Philippines headquarters and registered with the Department of Social Welfare and Development. I was sent to an orientation session for volunteers, to have my work explained to me.

I was confused within minutes. Was it jet-lag? I kept staring at the PowerPoint, thinking "I should be understanding this," but the presenter wasn't making sense. I guess I was jet-lagged because it took me a few minutes to realize that while the PowerPoint was written in English, the presenter was speaking in Filipino. Not wishing to cause anyone extra work, I focused on the slides, smiled when the rest of the Filipino-speaking volunteers did ("Good joke, Madame Presenter!") and then we were split into groups. The problem was, I had no idea what we were supposed to do in those groups. So I went up to the presenter and asked her if I could get a briefing in English. Sometimes it's best to ask questions — even though, let it be known, that I *hate* to ask questions or for directions. She led me on a tour of the humanitarian relief base — warehouse after warehouse stacked with raw food goods — ingredients that I would help prepare into meals for those in need.

Finally, we plopped ourselves down at a line of tables and she introduced me to the rest of the assembly line — all locals. There must have been a few hundred school groups and youth organizations as well as corporate employees working there that night — what an incredible team-building activity. I was placed on the coffee line which was added to the "gift package" for displaced families, consisting of rice, corned beef, sardines, noodles, and chopped meat. Our team prepared 1,200 family packs. I finally returned to the hotel around 2 am. Quite an arrival day!

The next morning began with a tour of the Jewish community and a briefing on the history of Filipino Jewry. The story is surprising, mostly because for me it was unexpected. My image of the Philippines is as one of the most overtly, passionately Catholic countries on the planet — they have an annual festival in which enthusiastic folk volunteer to be crucified (briefly and non-fatally, but still) to bring themselves closer to Jesus. Turns out that, while Catholicism is the vast majority religion, there have been Jews here since the 16th century. When the Spanish Inquisition drove Jews out of Spain, a community of Sephardim moved to the Northern Samar region of the Philippines, which at the time was a Spanish colony. Most were crypto-Jews, forced to practice their religion in secret since the Spanish rulers there would not allow it openly.

Usually, the story of Judaism in far-flung countries is more organic and less focused on individuals, but in the Philippines this is not the case. The first openly Jewish settlement began with three brothers, the Levy family, who emigrated from Alsace-Lorraine in 1870, after the Franco-Prussian War. Levy Hermanos, as their companies were called, became a business empire, covering gem import, jewelry making, pharmaceuticals, and even, much later, automobiles. Another Alsatian Jew, Leopold Kahn, held such lofty roles as president of the French Chamber of Commerce and the consul-general of France to the Philippines. The Suez Canal had opened in 1869, which led to far easier international trade, and Jewish communities followed in the Philippines, moving there from Turkey, Egypt, and Syria. Still, the community there was limited to less than one-hundred people (influential though they were) until the Spanish-American War led to the Philippines coming under the control of the United States, which then permitted the open practice of Judaism. Scores of American Jewish soldiers, having served in the Spanish-American War, remained in the Philippines. They were followed by a group of Thomasites, 600 American teacher volunteers who moved from the US aboard a ship called *Thomas* (hence their nickname) to establish a public school system in the Philippines. The US government funded this to the tune of $105,000 at the time — over $3 million in today's money. While the Thomasites were a diverse group, hailing from 192 different educational institutions (including Harvard, Yale, and Cornell), many were Jewish. The Philippines has them to thank for their modern educational system.

Manila, the capital of the Philippines, was also a safe place for Jewish refugees from Europe during the Philippine Commonwealth period (1935–

1946), welcoming Jews both from Europe, escaping fascism, and those who had already come to Asia, such as the lively Shanghai Jewish community which felt endangered when the Japanese occupied Beijing in 1937. Officially, 1,300 Jewish refugees from Europe arrived between 1937 and 1941.

One of the great benefits of my extensive travels has been to learn stories of Jews in places that one might not associate with them. The Philippines was the biggest surprise for me, of all the countries I've visited.

At an Air Force base in Manila, I saw cargo planes landing, dropping off people who had been rescued. Families looking for their relatives would wait on the tarmac, eyes rising in hope each time a new plane would land. I tried to help the local volunteers distribute clothes, food, and water, and also tried to arrange for some temporary housing for those displaced.

Part of my approach is asking questions and listening when someone felt the need to speak to a sympathetic soul, even if he were a stranger in a yarmulke. One woman I spoke to looked up at me and simply said, "I'm sorry, I can't talk now. I'm still in mourning. I lost six family members."

All I could do was try to be empathetic. I replied, "I'm so sorry to hear that." I thought that might be all she was up for, but she continued speaking for a few minutes. Speaking to a sympathetic human, regardless of who they are, can bring relief, siphoning off the pressure pent up inside.

I spotted a young girl carrying a violin. That haunts me to this day. You think to yourself, if you have to suddenly leave your home, what do you take with you? I'd take a passport, my laptop, my personal papers …. This adolescent girl took what I suppose was most valuable to her: a violin.

From there I went to Pasay City, where I was asked to spread the word about volunteer opportunities across the country and share them through call-ins and via social media. Following a couple of business meetings in the late afternoon, I was afforded a unique and very special opportunity. I was given a list of found survivors of the typhoon and contact information of the loved ones in search of them. I felt honored to be the bringer of good news in such a time of turmoil and anxiety. I was asked to call them and advise their families that these people, lost in the storm, had been found alive. Tears of joy were heard throughout the night, and some were mine. But I was also keenly aware that someone else had been tasked with making the opposite sort of phone call — the news that a body had been found. It put things into stark perspective.

Aisa from Tacloban had been one of the first evacuees to Manila and was working alongside me that night. She told me how she had found out, only 48 hours earlier, that her mother, who she thought had perished, was alive, although very hungry and waiting to be evacuated. The most moving story for me was of Caramen from Leyte, who was looking for her brother — she'd been told that he was dead. Now I had information in front of me that he was alive, but I'd been given nothing but an address and the source of information. Now Caramen was on the phone with me. I asked her to hold, and I contacted a third party, her brother, so we patched through a homemade conference call: I held the speaker of one phone to the receiver of the other and heard screams of happiness and relief. I knew that the mission was accomplished.

After about 30 hours in the storm center — where Typhoon Haiyan (Yolanda) had affected nearly fifteen million people killing 4,000 and displacing around two million, there were moments and stories of joy amongst the tragedy and sadness. One of the most heartwarming stories that I heard was that of a blind Filipino woman who visited the Israeli Field Hospital in Bogo. After a two-hour surgery, she experienced light for the first time. As a practicing Jew, I have always tried to live according to the laws given to my people by example "as a light unto the Nation." Here was an example of this metaphor made literal.

Now came my time to take that first taxi driver's advice and set out for Tacloban, where he'd said they could use help more than anywhere else.

As a tourism professional, I know how valuable specificity and reliability are to travelers. My flight to Tacloban was an example of what my clients dread. I couldn't figure out when the flight actually left. My ticket said one time, the website said another, and no one was picking up the phone at the airport. So I played it safe and set out at 2 am.

Once at the airport, it was clear that I wasn't the only one in doubt. The flight seemed to be composed of passengers of more nationalities than countries I'd visited, no one quite sure when to be there, so all arrived as early as possible. They were each going for different reasons — journalists, medical, United Nations, recovery efforts, insurance adjusters, spiritual leaders, volunteers, and locals in search of family — but all from abroad and here to help.

While I had been in contact with the Philippine Red Cross before leaving Manila, they hadn't been able to tell me exactly what to do and where to go when I landed. Very uncharacteristically of me, this time I was cool with this. Had I been on vacation, then the flight departure time confusion, and uncertainty about where to go when I landed would have driven me nuts. But knowing that I was in the midst of a country in crisis, recognizing that I wanted to ease their burden, not add to it in any way, however minor, my neuroses agreed to recede. I would figure out on my own what to do once there if I couldn't find anyone to instruct me. No big whoop. Easy-peasy. (Note: I'm the farthest thing from "easy-peasy" in all other moments of life, but Volunteer Stuart manages to channel his inner chill).

Tacloban is a provincial capital with a population of a quarter million, some 360 miles from Manila. It had been the capital of the Philippines during a period of the Commonwealth Government — the one that had so openly helped European Jews escape fascism. But much of the city was destroyed during Typhoon Haiyan, when a thirteen-foot storm surge rammed through it on November 8, 2013. A US Marine on-site was quoted as saying, "I don't believe there is a single structure that is not destroyed or severely damaged in some way — every single building, every single house." Previous incarnations of the city had similarly been wiped away by typhoons, in 1897 and 1912. This was an ever-present danger, living so close to so wild an ocean.

With no phone or internet connection upon arrival in Tacloban, the Red Cross was unable to reach me. No problem: I went with a Plan B. After a quick donning of tallit and tefillin in what was left of their airport — basically tar pavement and rubble amidst tents — I completed an abridged morning prayer service (I usually do the full daily prayers every day), which drew the stares of many a passer-by. I set off for the nearest tent city, but I couldn't see any volunteers at work. So I started walking into town.

On the way, I met a young man who wanted to hear about my "Muslim life." I liked his friendly curiosity, but I tried to explain to him I'm actually not Muslim, but Jewish. He nodded that he understood, then asked why I wore "a Muslim hat?"

"No, this is a yarmulke, a ... well, uh, a Jewish hat."

He nodded that he understood but was clearly only further confused. No matter, he invited me to his roadside tent, where we chatted for a bit before I said that I wanted to go to town to see the hospital. He told me that we could walk the eight kilometers, or he could get me a "tricycle." I had visions of me, a grown man wearing a "Muslim hat," riding a children's tricycle eight kilometers into town. "Sure, why not," I said, figuring I should do as the locals.

He nodded but warned that it would be expensive since tricycles run on diesel and diesel was in short supply and everything was about ten times what it normally cost. Now I was really curious to see a tricycle running on diesel, cost be damned.

Turns out "tricycle" meant "motorcycle." My driver, Roel, was without question the highlight of my day.

He asked me which hospital I wanted to go to and what was wrong with me.

I told him I was healthy and just wanted to visit some of the people who had been hurt in the typhoon to offer whatever solace I could to them. He noted my headgear and asked if I was a rabbi (a better guess than Mr. Tricycle). I said that I was not, but I was Jewish.

Driving by his church, we got into a religious exchange and that's when he truly began to open up. He told me about November 8, when the typhoon landed on the shores of Tacloban. They had known for a week that it was coming, but the general public hadn't expected it to be as serious as it was. When it approached land, he put his family of five into his "tricycle" and they drove to the church. He said that he couldn't see anything and, to the best of his recollection, he rode in neutral the entire way, as the wind just blew them along. They arrived at the church and, together with other "brothers" and "sisters," they climbed to the highest place possible, keeping the children ahead of them.

The water levels kept rising and roofs were blown off. They prayed for their safety and, at the same time, said goodbye to one another. Fortunately, Roel's entire family survived, as did everyone that was in the church with them during the storm.

It was a beautiful thing. Regardless of whether you believe that their survival was divine intervention, luck, or a smart move, Roel and the congregation felt comfort in prayer in a time of terror. That's one of the best things religion can do, soothe us in the face of death. It doesn't matter at all which religion you choose or whom you pray to.

As we drove through town, he would stop every couple of minutes, and not only because of traffic, which was slowed due to only one lane being in operation, due in turn to the masses of rubble still crowding the road. No, he stopped so often to get off the "tricycle" and hug someone. With each stop, he'd just tell me that he was thankful they were alive, as he hadn't known until he spotted them on the road. The losses were that fresh. This was repeated continuously throughout the morning.

I saw many things that stayed with me on this trip. I vividly recall the many mothers carrying their babies on their backs, and not only infants, even three-year-olds. People were literally carrying their lives with them, sometimes with nothing left but the clothes they were wearing, their family members (if they hadn't been lost), and perhaps a duffel or even just a garbage bag of possessions.

We finally arrived at Bethany Hospital, which was largely set up in the field adjacent to the damaged hospital proper. In addition to the locals, there were forty medical teams from around the world there volunteering and helping. While the first wave after the typhoon was triaging injuries from falling debris and the like, the issue at hand now was preventing the spread of disease. There was also a mass immunization project underway to protect against measles, polio, and tetanus, all of which were still major problems there. The focus was on vaccinating the 1.4 million children displaced from their homes by the typhoon.

This was a familiar situation for me. I manage to get myself to a crisis zone, but I'm there unofficially, so I'm on my own to figure out how to help. I don't want to add work to the volunteers who already have their hands full, so I just get to it, improvising anything that looks like it might do some good.

I spotted some children huddled together and looking unhappy. Roel said that they were probably orphans. I saw a pile of books, but the only ones in English were a Grolier Encyclopedia and an ancient *Highlights* magazine. I grabbed them anyway, sat beside the five children, and started reading to them.

Roel had sent his family to Cebu, the second largest city in the Philippines, right after the storm. While it would be best for his family there, a city that was also damaged but nowhere near as badly, he wasn't leaving. He said Tacloban was his home, and he would rebuild, then bring his family back. He felt an obligation to stay there with his "brothers" and keep the church as a haven and place to pray.

As we headed to the house where he was staying, along with a number of his brothers — I wasn't sure if they were actually his brothers or his "brothers"

— he mentioned offhandedly to me, "Oh another dead body." We passed one along the road. He said that, in the days immediately after the typhoon, there were hundreds of corpses along the side of the road, just washed up. Actually, he used much more descriptive language, but I won't repeat it here. They were all cleaned up now, he said, well, almost. Thrown onto a truck so they could try to identify them when the families came back. But most would end up in a mass grave. He spoke without emotion as if this were merely a fact of life. I wondered if this was a Philippine stoicism or just Roel, or whether he was now inured to this but was fighting emotions inside.

He took me to his house, or rather where his house used to be. It was just a pile of rubble. Despite this, one of his neighbors guards the area, as they're afraid of looting. His wife wants him to save whatever he can but he says he hasn't found anything. He's trying to find his children's birth certificates and some photos. He shrugs. "The only thing I saved was my family, my tricycle, and the clothes I was wearing."

He wears the same thing every day, as new clothing hasn't yet been distributed. He said that he was embarrassed to attend church always in the same clothes, but figured G-d would understand. We moved on to his temporary residence, at the home of his brother (without quotation marks) and his brother's family.

I try to adhere to local traditions, out of respect, and follow the lead of my host. So when he removed his shoes upon entering, I did the same. Then he removed his socks, so I did the same. Then he took off his shirt — I suppose to wash it. Here I felt guilty but didn't follow suit.

He introduced me to his brother's five children, ranging in age from two to twelve. They didn't know where Israel was, so I showed them on a map in a world atlas they kept in the house. I asked them if they wanted to learn some Hebrew, so we made a deal — they'd teach me some Filipino and I'd teach them a few words of Hebrew.

Roel then offered me some rice and beans. The generosity of these people, who didn't know when their next meal would arrive, astonished me. I politely declined. Normally I know that accepting an offer of a meal is considered good manners, but I couldn't bring myself to do so, knowing the straits they were navigating — not to mention that it wasn't kosher.

At the end of the day, he took me back to the airport to check in for my return flight to Manila. When we got there, I wanted to pay him, but he refused to take the money. I didn't know how to make him, but there was no way it was going back into my pocket. So I improvised (Planner Stuart can, in fact, improvise when circumstance requires). Most uncharacteristic of me, I took the shirt off my back and told him to wear this to church when he goes tonight. That he agreed to. I then told him I wanted him to give the money to the church to feed those who couldn't feed themselves. That was the clincher. We both parted ways, content.

I find myself trying to recall stories of those whose lives were ravaged by disaster, whether refugees or typhoon victims, in order to tell their stories, to give them a voice. I'm usually telling it to friends and congregations. I've often written informal articles, for instance for *The Times of Israel* (in which earlier versions of some of the stories here first appeared). I think there's value in that. Simply telling the story so the names of the voiceless won't be forgotten. It's what Hamlet tells Laertes to do at the end of the play. It's one of the reasons why I'm writing this book and including so many stories of those I encountered.

I often ask myself why I'm driven to travel the world, not just for pleasure but so many of my early travels to help my new homeland, Israel, and later, to volunteer in the wake of disasters.

For the Philippines, at least, I had a sense of wanting to pay back the good that the country had done for my people. The one aspect of the story of Judaism in the Philippines that I had known related to the Second World War. Then-President Manuel L. Quezon and the people of the Philippines did what no other country had the moral and ethical courage to do — they opened the door to potentially 10,000 Jewish refugees from Austria and Germany. They received 1,300 European Jewish refugees between 1937 and December 1941 when the Japanese invasion reached Manila. President Quezon openly condemned the Nazi persecution of our people — something no other leader had the guts to do, so overtly.

But why do I do it? Aren't there enough people on the ground there? What is someone like me, non-emergency personnel, going to be able to do, anyway? Don't think that I didn't ponder these questions every time I set out, whether to Greece, or Nepal, or the Philippines, or Long Island.

My first instinct was always to offer myself to an official group that was already at the site, and which has the infrastructure to make a difference on a big scale. But for each crisis area, after a quick look and knowing the bureaucratic channels that are often obstacles for those making such attempts, I decided to "pay back" on my own. There was somehow more meaning in going solo. I hope that my admittedly compulsive do-gooding will encourage others, maybe even you, as you read this, no matter where in the world they are today, to do one more thing for the benefit of humankind tomorrow.

In 1940, President Quezon said, "It is my hope and indeed my expectation that the people of the Philippines will have in the future every reason to be glad when the time of need came their country extended a hand of welcome." It is always, every day, our turn to extend our hand and help those in a time of need. As we would hope to have a hand extended to us when our time comes.

At the airport, on my way home, a woman approached me. She said that she was blessed because she'd seen two Jews in one week! I hadn't spotted anyone else who I could identify as a Jew. I'm pretty sure that she had seen me twice in one week — the yarmulke gave it away. But it was a lovely thing to hear that this Catholic Filipino woman should take spotting two Jews in one week as a sign of blessing.

Chapter 13

Transformational Travel is a Thing

Volunteer Nomadism

I will speak that I may find relief; for there is a redemptive quality for an agitated mind in the spoken word, and a tormented soul finds peace in confessing.

— Rabbi Joseph B. Sloveitchik

That trip to the Philippines changed me. Look, travel changes people, inevitably for the better. It's nothing new to say this, but it is worth spending some time considering.

Transformation through travel, personal growth through journeys, is a literary typology. Odysseus would not have been the same had he not been forced by the wills of the gods to wind his way back from Troy, home to Ithaca, over many years and adventures. The Israelites were bound to wander the desert for forty years after the Exodus from Egypt. Buddha walked throughout what is now India. Jack Kerouac's *On the Road* crisscrossed America by car in search of a more mundane, personal version of enlightenment. Even such popular memoirs as Elizabeth Gilbert's *Eat, Pray, Love* follow an author who feels lost and finds herself through travel. The oldest of all known literary works, *The Epic of Gilgamesh,* written over 4,000 years ago, follows the Babylonian king as he travels to the "edges of the Earth" in search of the secret of eternal life — not finding it, he returns home, for the journey did bring him peace, accepting his own mortality. Transformational journeys are an inbuilt part of the human experience, whether true stories or those mapped out in fiction.

But most of those are quests. The protagonist travels to reach somewhere, to do something, at which point they return home, with the understanding that home is where they prefer to be. The journey-as-quest is necessary, not desired.

What if the journey itself is all we need? No quest required, no end point, no dragon to slay, no magical ingredient to retrieve. There are such travelers, too. Voluntary nomads, as they sometimes like to call themselves. Some live on the sea, in boats that function as an always-mobile home base. Others are literally backpacking through life, like Americans Mike and Anne Howard, who set out on their honeymoon in January 2012 and never stopped, eventually turning their blog, HoneyTrek, into a source of income, and appearing in the media wherever they went as the couple on an endless honeymoon. They have no "home" and live entirely out of backpacks that qualify as carry-on luggage. They've been to sixty-three countries and counting. They never plan to stop.

There are those of us who feel compelled to travel. The term "wanderlust" is the desire to travel. It comes from the Old English word, *wandrian,* which meant "to move about aimlessly." The destination is not the purpose. Movement is.

Inevitably literary versions of epic journeys conclude that their real journey has taken place within. But so often physical movement, the being elsewhere, the encounter of new things, the break from the quotidian, is required to prompt inner change. The compulsion to travel can derive from an adventurous curiosity, the desire to see new things, to push human boundaries. Or it can be an expression of an inner disquiet, an escape from the status quo, which is easier to distance yourself from if you are actually in motion.

Which of these defines my desire to travel? It is most likely a combination of factors, in me and in any of us. Perhaps it's for the psychologists to decide what I feel compelled to move away from when I travel.

I certainly feel a proper compulsion to travel in aid of crises. I'm the first to admit that I'm no saint — I travel for crisis volunteer work because it makes me feel good (or at least better) in that I can help others. It is not entirely selfless, but maybe it's a more expansive reason than if I were to travel just to check boxes off a bucket list or to test the ten tallest bungee jumps in the world (which, by now you'll know, isn't my style).

It's a reasonable question to ask yourself: Why do I travel? Which destinations call to me? Do I travel only to reach specific locations — given the Star Trek option to be "beamed" instantly to the location, would I prefer it? Or is the entire package: anticipation, packing, the trip to the airport or other primary mode of transport, the flight (the movies on a small screen, the tiny bags of peanuts — when it's not a nut-free flight — the squishy double-pronged headphones), the landing, the orientation, the hotel check-in — are those all elements that contribute beneficially to the whole? Do I want experiences or sites or relaxation? Some of us, those who feel overworked, might travel to a single spot to lounge and unwind, with as little to think about as possible once we're there. Others are sightseers. We want to see X, Y, and Z, so we journey to those sights. Experiences are a newer category, answering the question many vacationers have: I'm here, so what can I do here that I cannot do back home?

Many would say that they travel to create memories. There's something to that. For millennia, the "art of memory," *ars memoriae,* was taught. Memorization techniques were necessary before computers got so accessible that they could fit in our pockets, and our smartphones could look up and recall anything we liked. The famous mathematician and philosopher, Giordano Bruno, earned his keep traveling to princely courts in Renaissance Europe, teaching memorization techniques. Understanding a bit about how we humans remember things helps us understand why we travel to "create" memories. It's not that we cannot remember things from daily life at home. But the main takeaway is that we tend to forget, or gloss over, what we're used to. If you journey to northern Norway to see the Aurora Borealis, and it's likely a once-in-a-lifetime experience, you'll remember it more vividly, appreciate it more, than if you live in northern Norway and see it many times a year, over the course of decades.

We humans best remember what surprises us, what is new, what provokes strong emotion (joy, despair, hilarity, jealousy, anger, gratitude), and what is surreal. The weird, the bizarre, stands out because it is so *different* from what we're used to. Our minds play a trick on us when it comes to repetitive activities that are normal and every day for us. We can remember them, but they tend to blend into a single memory. Were we to play chess just once with one of our children, we'd remember it more crisply than if we played daily for years. The weekday walks to work all merge into an amorphous single memory — aside from those outlier days, when a pigeon took great liberties on your head, or you nearly got run over by a bicyclist, or you happened to meet your future wife.

The Czech novelist, Milan Kundera, wrote a novel called *Slowness* that addresses just this. The plot revolves around a pair of lovers who become aware that they can only spend a single day more with one another before separating forever. To make the day spread out and feel like a rich, expansive series of memories when they look back on it later on, they plan as diverse an array of experiences as they can. Each is like a chapter in the day, and each will be better preserved in memory than if they were to spend the whole day doing just one thing.

With this in mind, we can in fact plan "making memories" by planning activities that will be far from our daily routine, whatever that might be. Surprising, new, bizarre, surreal sites, activities, tastes, vistas, experiences will each crystallize into vivid memories that we can happily recall when we're back home from our travels. By going elsewhere, we anticipate more differences from the home routine. So it's easier to "make memories" by traveling to them, than by trying to introduce novelties into our own living rooms.

Most of this memory-making happens by happenstance. We experience things, particularly those surprises, and they stick. Some of them are so vivid, new, thought-provoking, moving, special that they transform how we think of ourselves or the world around us. These moments are precious but unplanned.

But how many of us consciously travel to change, fundamentally, who we are, or at least our outlook on life and on ourselves?

There is now a catchphrase in the industry called "transformational travel." It refers to journeys that fundamentally change the journeyer. That can happen even if it is unplanned. It can be most effective when it comes as a surprise. That sunset over the Indian Ocean, your glimpse of the mosaic on Torcello, the taste of Neapolitan pizza, the spread of Aurora Borealis over Tromso, the rhinoceros and her baby you photographed on safari, the conversation with a stranger over a pint in a remote pub near Galway.

But now there are companies that will help clients map out a journey, with the plan that it *will* be transformational. A sort of pilgrimage within oneself. It could feel artificial, deciding that, "If I do X, then I'll feel Y." Forcing oneself into enlightenment.

I'll climb Kilimanjaro.

I'll scuba dive with manta rays off the Australian coast.

I'll run the Berlin marathon.

I'll walk the Great Wall of China.

I'll do a yoga retreat in Sri Lanka.

I'll cuddle a panda.

Actually, all of those sound pretty good. Here's the thing: as dismissive as we may wish to be about such things, they do work. It's really about setting a goal, preparing for it, looking forward to it, physically and geographically moving beyond your everyday orbit, achieving a predetermined goal, feeling satisfied and self-actualized, then returning home to reflect on it. It's a recipe, but recipes produce the best dishes.

Where does my own travel fit into all this? Wanderlust is an inherent part of me. In all honesty, the idea of visiting one hundred countries (out of 198 or so on Earth) came to me only in recent years, when I tallied up where I'd been and realized that I wasn't so far from the century mark. Maybe I could reach it by age sixty? Then the pandemic slowed me down but reaching a round one hundred still seems feasible and like a good goal. But it's a target not about itself, but something that occurred to me organically because of my love for traveling. I don't hunt destinations, I hunt journeys. And while I do go sightseeing, I'm not particularly ravenous when it comes to must-see places, nor am I very adventurous, when it comes to adrenaline (which I prefer to keep under control) and food (traveling the world kosher doesn't permit wild experimentation). I'm not seeking memories, or selfies in front of famous monuments. I don't feel the need to find enlightenment because my Jewish faith fulfills me. My spiritual side is in order. So I'm left with the journeys themselves, for the sake of journeying. The idea of hitting one-hundred countries was merely an afterthought, a guiding superstructure to what I've already been doing my whole life.

TRAVEL THERAPY

In anticipation of my "century" of countries, number one-hundred, I posted on Facebook of my impending trip to Bulgaria.

Traveling has always been my ultimate passion, and let me tell you, I take my hobbies seriously. Ten years ago, I reached the pinnacle of wanderlust achievement by visiting my fiftieth state, the elusive North Dakota. I know, I know, everyone's clamoring to get there—it's a must-see on every travel enthusiast's bucket list! As my kids said, at least it won't be our fiftieth!

But as I stood there, gazing at the majestic North Dakotan landscape, plopping mezuzot on any doorpost that would accept, I thought to myself, "Hey, why stop at fifty states? Why not aim for something truly ambitious?" And that's when it hit me like a suitcase falling from an overhead bin: I should visit one hundred countries before I turn sixty! It seemed like a stellar idea at the time, but little did I know what I was getting myself into.

Fast forward to a couple of months ago, when I triumphantly landed in Bermuda, country number ninety-nine. The finish line was in sight, and I could almost taste the victory. I had hoped that my entire family could join me for the grand finale, the one-hundredth country, but alas, scheduling conflicts are the mortal enemy of every family vacation plan. We just couldn't find a date when we could all go together. So, in a moment of sheer spontaneity and borderline insanity, I decided to take matters into my own hands.

This week, I will find myself with Carol and Dafna in the beautiful land of Bulgaria. I'm on the cusp of achieving my daring goal.

That's right, this Shabbat, I'll be celebrating my travel triumph in the country that will etch my name into the annals of adventure. Why Bulgaria, you may ask? Well, let's just say it was a whimsical choice driven by a mixture of sheer determination and a desperate need for a vacation from planning family vacations.

Now, the journey to reach this momentous destination has been no less than an adventure of epic proportions. The tales of my escapades, the mishaps, the close calls with missed flights, cancelled flights, rude passengers from historic lands and lost passports—they're all worthy of their own travel documentary series. But fear not, I promise to regale you with those anecdotes another time. Stay tuned, because next week, I'll be back with more thrilling tales from the travel trenches. Trust me, you won't want to miss it!

I didn't want to miss my own hundredth, either, and it turned out to be trickier to achieve than I'd thought. That line I jokingly penned about a suitcase falling from an overhead bin proved all too portentous.

Even for a veteran traveler like me, mishaps can (mis)happen. On my way from a conference via various stops Bulgaria to score my hundredth country, a flight was delayed. Someone had opened the emergency exit, releasing the slide. It took three hours to get this sorted, repaired, and the plane checked and ready for takeoff. This made me miss my connecting flight. I was booked on another flight, and all might have been well, but we wound up sitting on the plane for another three hours, unable to take off due to thunderstorms, but also not deplaning, as the airport hoped to get us up and away should the storm pass by. Multiple delays meant that the crew timed out—their maximum legal shift was over, and a new crew had to replace them. It was 1:30am by then, when they sent us off the plane and back to the gate.

This sounds like a moment when the airline would be obliged to provide hotel rooms for the passengers, but the airline reps said no, they wouldn't do that because the delay was weather-related, and so it was just bad luck, not their responsibility.

I would have none of that. I wouldn't have been on the storm-delayed plane had my previous flight not been delayed due to a mechanical issue, fixing the emergency exit. It took an hour for them to accept responsibility for putting me up, so I collapsed in a free hotel room around 2:30am. Just long enough to shower and make it back to the airport at 5am for the replacement of the replacement flight. This was more about principal—I didn't absolutely need two hours of hotel room and a meal voucher, but I was inconvenienced and entitled to this, and it didn't feel right to be told otherwise. The lesson is that you need to know your rights as a passenger, and stand up for them, as no one else will do it for you and airlines look for any reason not to incur extra costs.

On one of my connections on the way to Bulgaria made the warning to "Be careful when opening the overhead bins, as objects may have shifted during flight" unfortunately accurate. I opened the overhead bin upon landing, and out fell my backpack. I didn't think much of this at the time, just glad it didn't smack anyone in the head on the way down to the floor. But when I had deplaned and pulled my laptop out of the backpack, I saw that the screen had cracked and it wouldn't turn on.

Now, any time of year is a busy time for me, and my laptop is my primary tool: for working, for communication. I need a laptop at all times, and I need my laptop, full of my files. I remained calm, a reaction which certainly surprised me (and by now, I imagine will surprise you). There was nowhere in the airport to buy a new laptop. I was trying to figure out what to do, and made the radical decision of flying without a laptop to work on during the flight.

This wasn't so bad. I actually slept on the plane and arrived refreshed. Maybe this could be a thing? Nah, I want my laptop.

I wound up contacting Dafna and asking her to bring a spare laptop from home. So, on to Bulgaria!

When I arrived at the hotel, there was a cake waiting for me, covered in chocolate and emblazoned with a large "100" in icing (as well as an even larger Hyatt Regency medallion—never miss a branding opportunity). I like the idea that my renown preceded me, but more likely my family called ahead to let the staff know that this was a special trip.

It would be narratively satisfying if I did something unique for my century of countries visited. Get a tattoo of a world map or something like that. But by now you know me well enough to know that the big celebration would entail visiting local points of Jewish interest and acquiring a Starbucks mug.

Carol and I went to the old synagogue in Sofia, Bulgaria, which was consecrated in 1909 and is the third largest in Europe. We go to synagogues wherever we go, both to take a look and also to attend services whenever possible. We visited other synagogues in Bulgaria and, to my surprise, at one we ran into someone I knew. This man had called me once for support for his daughter a few months earlier. It was an astonishing coincidence, and underscored how the volunteer work we do can touch people we might assume we'd never meet, or never meet again. But fate, if you want to call it that, or G-d, works in mysterious ways. The world is smaller than any of us realize, a further reason to extend kindness and compassion to anyone seeking it, wherever they may be.

But synagogues are not our only tradition. We also visit Starbucks wherever in the world we happen to be—and, inevitably, there's a Starbucks to be found, from Aspen to Zürich. Carol has a vast mug collection, over sixty. We'll always get a Starbucks mug, whether together or, if I'm traveling on my own to a new country, it's the go-to souvenir I'll bring home to her. And so it was with nation one-hundred.

It's a safer bet as a gift than a live Moldovan chicken.

There are some through-lines that I can spot, beyond synagogues and Starbucks mugs. I'm interested in seeing how Jews live and survive in vastly different countries and cultures with limited Jewish populations. I like the mechanics of travel, of sorting things out, finding hotels, booking transport — I'm a travel professional, after all, so traveling is my busman's holiday. I feel better about myself when I travel to help others. They may be essentially locals, like my fellow Israelis, or former neighbors, like those who suffered after Hurricane Sandy. Or, they may be complete strangers from vastly different worlds than mine, as in the Philippines or Syrian refugees in Greece or Nepal (as we'll see next). Humans in need are humans. I've also more recently grown interested in seeing how mental healthcare is tackled in each country I visit.

So my personal approach becomes:

Travel (while keeping kosher) + Volunteering + Exploring Judaism + Improving (or Maintaining) My Mental Health = Stuart's Travel Recipe.

What I get out of it is, simply, feeling better than I otherwise would. It was not until very recently that I realized that, for years — decades, even — I've been clinically depressed. Travel alleviated this feeling.

It's worth considering what your personal recipe is. Few take the time to think about it, and it's a good exercise in self-understanding. For travel is something we can turn to for pleasure or temporary relief from whatever brings us down about our daily grind.

The thing is, wherever we go, there we are. There's no escaping our own minds. 15th-century theologian Thomas a Kempis wrote, "Wherever you go, you take yourself with you, and you will always find yourself."

This approach was updated by the doctor and specialist in stress reduction through mindfulness, Jon Kabat-Zinn, in his aptly titled *Wherever You Go There You Are*: "Perhaps the most 'spiritual' thing any of us can do is simply to look through our own eyes, see with eyes of wholeness, and act with integrity and kindness."

Chapter 14

Travel for Disaster Relief Work

Nepal

Emotional pain is not something that should be hidden away and never spoken about. There is truth in your pain, there is growth in your pain, but only if it's first brought out into the open.

— Steven Aitchison

Having gotten a taste of travel for volunteer work, the good it seemed to do, both in my helping others and, in doing so, helping myself, I was soon on my way to do whatever small part I could to offer aid in the wake of a new disaster. When I left Ben Gurion Airport on a Sunday night, headed to Nepal to help after a disastrous earthquake, the security agent said to me: "You should have a successful mission and return home safely." These words moved me. I hadn't really thought of myself as heading out on a mission. Instead, I was just offering a bit of help, whatever I could, letting those affected know that there was love and care for them outside of Nepal.

As I passed immigration, I saw a poster that I'd seen many times before.

It read: "Outside Israel – The Country is You! – Represent Us with Honor!" I always found it to be a nice and catchy message. But as I headed towards my gate, I thought: *this week that message will have real meaning, and I must do my best. Maybe I am on some kind of mission.*

Central Nepal was struck by a shattering earthquake on April 25, 2015. The quake registered a 7.9 magnitude on the Richter scale, and its epicenter was less than 100 km from Nepal's capital city of Kathmandu, and near other large cities, such as Pokhara — some *6.6 million* people reside within that devastating earthquake's epicenter.

The destruction created by the main quake and over twenty aftershocks, ranging from a 4.5 to 6.6 magnitude, was catastrophic. The effects were felt as far as India, Bangladesh, and China, and even led to a massive avalanche on Mt. Everest. More than 8,000 people were killed and approximately 18,000 injured. Hundreds of thousands were left homeless.

After the tragedy occurred, relief workers poured into Nepal. A poor but developing country, Nepal has been unable to recover from such massive destruction using its own resources alone. As the death toll and recovery costs swiftly rose, worldwide support followed. The single largest aid force came from Israel, a fact of which I am proud.

Knowing me, you won't be surprised to learn that I was among the volunteers. Disaster relief is my "silent" middle name. I feel it's the least I can do, but I also don't want to ever feel like I'm bragging about it, because that entirely defeats the purpose. I debated over whether to mention it in this book at all, but I think including it tells my story most completely and it is certainly a big part of me, and one I hope might encourage others. Guilt and sympathy are my propulsion, but I feel any good person should do all they can do to help those in need, whoever and wherever those in need may be.

My decision to come was a last-minute one. Instinct told me to hop on the first flight to Nepal, but I was both busy and fatigued. Still, my tendency is to put the well-being of others in need over my own. That sounds noble and I feel it is, but it can also get me into trouble.

Because of my previous experience with disaster relief logistics, largely learned from my experiences on the ground after the Philippines typhoon, I had received requests for assistance from several organizations. Although I provided some logistical help from afar, I decided to pass on traveling to Nepal in person. "Someone else will go," I told myself.

But my thoughts would not settle. So often we hear the phrase, "You only live once." The attitude I try to live by is: "I will only die once and want to live each and every day to the fullest." That is an easy mantra to say, but it is often hard to do. Little did I know, at the time, that these phrases would haunt me. At the time I felt, only subconsciously, the stirrings of the mental illness that I would only later realize I'd been living with for years. My desire to make my life useful to others, to people I didn't know, is a mark of goodwill but also a bit unusual. Looking back, I can see how it might have meant that I felt my life with my family didn't have enough meaning to it, that I felt a void within it that I tried to fill through repeated overt acts of humanitarian assistance.

Having done relief work in settings ranging from the Philippines to post-Hurricane Sandy New York, I wondered if I was the "someone" who *should* go. The words of Isaiah 6:8 came back to me: *"I heard the voice of the Lord, saying, Who shall I send, and who will go for us? Then said I, Here am I; send me."* But the Lord wasn't addressing anyone with a tourism business to run and four children to care for.

It wasn't until 3 pm on a Sunday that I finally made the decision to head out that very night. I ran to the store to get some food and threw some clothes in a bag. I was off!

The first leg of my journey began in Kathmandu. A city of 2.5 million inhabitants, Kathmandu is a metropolis I would have loved to visit under other circumstances, in my role as a travel professional. In 2013, Trip Advisor ranked Kathmandu as third among the top ten on-the-rise travel destinations worldwide. The entirety of the surrounding Kathmandu Valley was declared a UNESCO World Heritage site due to its plentiful medieval architecture.

An ancient city, Kathmandu is home to numerous palaces, temples, and historical museums, all against the magnificent backdrop of the Himalayas. While some of the city's treasures survived the recent quake, many historical sites were, sadly, part of the surrounding rubble.

I arrived at Kathmandu airport on Monday and immediately joined relief efforts there. First, I headed to Kathmandu Medical Teaching Hospital, near the airport. There, I assisted with distributing food to individuals who were searching for loved ones, hoping that they might show up at the hospital.

Next, I traveled to an emergency relief and distribution center, where supplies were being given out. Blankets and tents were provided to set up temporary shelters that those rendered homeless could set up in their own, now empty yards, or in one of the many tent cities lining the streets. Such tent cities served as temporary shelter for thousands of Nepal residents.

We volunteers also made and distributed "care packages" with available raw goods at the center. Their contents included rice, dry milk, coffee, chocolate, sugar, lentils, and beans. These precious supplies were distributed to family members waiting there for loved ones.

My last stop on Monday was at the Chabad House (Beit Chabad), which has done an amazing job in providing not only for all the Israelis in the area but also other quake survivors. There are a lot of Israeli Jews in Nepal, but they aren't permanent expats. It's a popular destination after completing one's army service, so Chabad House tends to cater to tourists or those there for extended (as in year-long) visits, rather than permanent immigrants. There, I dropped off food supplies that the Chabad Rabbi had requested from Israel. I also met with others to discuss how I might be able to help their efforts in the few days I would be in the country.

Before dawn on Tuesday, I left for the Village of Kakani, not far from Kathmandu. A scenic hour by car from the capital, the village is famed for its breathtaking views of the central and western Himalayas and the Ganesh Himal.

Two Indian nationals accompanied me to Kakani. These gentlemen were here for the same purpose I was — to deliver rice to hungry villagers. When I say "rice" I am not speaking about 2-lb. bags of rice from the local grocery store. Instead, we brought 25 kg bags (about fifty-five pounds each, less than my allotted seventy pounds per bag), enough to feed five or six families for an entire month.

At the crack of dawn, villagers lined up for the rice, each trying to get a bag for their own little cluster of family, friends, and survivors. This method reminded me of *moshavim*, Israel's cooperative agricultural settlements, where everyone has a very small plot of land to tend.

This spirit of cooperation was heartening to see, particularly in people who had gone through so much. Over 50% of the village was destroyed in the April 25th earthquake, but 100% of the locals were sleeping outside in tents because of damage to their homes. They feared that the unstable adobes would fall and injure them if they slept inside. Given the reality of aftershocks, such fear was not misplaced.

While in Kakani, I saw many injured villagers and heard story after story of what they had experienced. Some didn't find their loved ones for over forty-eight hours, while some never did.

After the rice distribution in Kakani, I headed back to Chabad House and reflected on everything I had seen in less than twenty-four hours. The contrast between the beautiful, serene Kathmandu Valley as it was less than three weeks prior, and the devastation I saw all around me was poignant, to say the least. Even more troubling were the faces of those I saw at every stop: visages dazed and flat, understandably so.

When I arrived at the Chabad House, I met with others to plan how best to contribute to a village rebuilding project. Then, I prepared to leave for the village of Bhaktapur, about thirty minutes from Kathmandu, where I was to help build temporary shelters.

Suddenly, the ground shook beneath me — and I realized I was in the middle of another earthquake.

In retrospect, through the act of writing about this especially, I can see my inner psychiatrist engaged in a bout of self-analysis. It's a fascinating act for anyone to engage in, writing about yourself, because it encourages a level of deep thought that otherwise our daily lives allow us to cruise past without giving it too much attention. I am a serial humanitarian assistance volunteer. There's a level of neurosis to the number of times I've flown around the world to help others. That's certainly a "good" habit to have, one that genuinely helps others, but the frequency with which I've done it, and the urgency I feel to do it, are compulsive. It's the work dysmorphia leading into what I dubbed philanthropic dysmorphia that I mentioned earlier. I'll read about a disaster somewhere around the world and I feel seized with a tremendous, forceful feeling that I should drop everything to go and help. I do feel a sense of worthiness when I'm helping people. It boosts my normally very low self-esteem. So it's a mutually beneficial compulsion, but still, compulsions are problematic. I suffer from a self-inflicted level of stress prior to embarking on a humanitarian mission — the feeling that I should or even must go is counterbalanced by my work, obligations to my own family, the cost involved, and so on. I'm essentially opting into making my life supremely more complicated than it was before, in order to help people. That's a good thing, but I'm doing it so much that I begin to wonder if it's an elaborate, subconscious attempt to gloss over my unhappiness in the at-home routine.

Helping others is a great rationalization to fly around the globe. But, as the cliché goes, you can travel all you like, but you can't escape yourself. If my issues are within me, then no amount of mileage and no number of volunteer projects will make me go away.

Still, I found temporary relief from all this while volunteering. It was afterward that the guilt about not having done enough would sink its teeth into me. While in the field, I had to focus on the problems before me, and so my dysmorphia receded. So I threw myself, as I always did, into my boots-on-the-ground work.

As I met with various individuals and organizations that week to discuss the logistics of the rebuilding plan, several important points were identified — and which might stand as a template for volunteers elsewhere and in the future.

First of all, the newly constructed homes should be safe and meet the needs of this Third World population. Many village families lived "off the grid," and did not strive for any deluxe accommodations, but merely what would be comfortable, safe, and secure.

Secondly, rather than "gifting" homes to the residents, I feel it important that they contribute. Instead of being treated as helpless, they will then have an active stake in building their futures in their damaged homeland. The goal was to build each home for around $7,000–10,000 with any additional expenses borne by the residents themselves. Most of them would receive some compensation from the government, but it could be a long bureaucratic process. Up to 90% of the expenses would be covered eventually by a combination of the Nepalese government and volunteer organizations.

My role in this endeavor began in Chilime. Lying in the Bagmati Zone of northern Nepal, Chilime is classified as a village development committee. Its purpose is to provide structure to village people at a local level and build community and public sector partnerships. Adding to their problems, a major hydroelectric plant located there was damaged in the quake, along with a dam that had been under construction. Many villagers were homeless. Following the devastation, a coordinated effort was going to be critical to restoring the quality of life for locals. Having a safe roof over their heads was an important start.

After a tour of the village, I returned to the outskirts of Kathmandu, where I had the opportunity to chat with displaced residents. My goal there was just to offer them an ear, some sympathy, and perhaps some hope. Sometimes just having another human being be there for you, giving you their attention, listening to your plight, can do a world of good. While many residents of the capital city can speak some degree of English, a more fluent local accompanied me. With his assistance, I heard many fascinating stories of survival.

Bishal is a tour guide who was leading a trek on Mt. Everest during the first earthquake. He managed to survive the resulting avalanche and was found after five days. Unfortunately, two of his trekkers were not so lucky. Bishal returned to his family in Kathmandu only to find his home destroyed and his family living in a tent. Bishal's passion is guiding, but he was fearful that there wouldn't be any trekkers here for a long time. He expressed his concern that he may need to find something else to do to help support his family.

Shirisha was seventeen at the time and spoke English fluently. She was graduating high school this year and has dreams of going to university in India. Shirisha hopes to become a doctor someday. In talking to this young lady, I could not help but think of my own 17-year-old daughter, Dafna, back home, and the stark contrasts of their lives. Shirisha was fascinated to learn that I was from Israel and kept saying how wonderful the people of Israel are (which is always music to my ears). Shirisha's parents had a shop in the Thamel section of Kathmandu and had met many Israelis. I had some extra Sderot T-shirts, each printed with a heart logo, with me, so I gave her one. Her face brightened with happiness, making me wish I had brought more.

Birsha was crying as we approached her tent. Given the circumstances, asking her what was wrong didn't seem appropriate. Instead, we offered her water and crackers and asked if we could sit. Birsha asked if we were reporters and seemed relieved when I said no. Then I told her that I was just a caring citizen of the world who came to do what little I could and that I planned to take messages back from anyone I might meet and to encourage others to help. "Oh, like the Red Crescent!" she exclaimed, probably thinking of the Red Cross. I reiterated that I was here on my own. She asked where I was from, and I said, "Israel."

"Oh, the army," she replied.

"No," I explained. "The Israeli Army was here, but I came on my own as they left, to be with the people of Nepal."

Understanding dawned. Birsha smiled and gave me a hug. Those who know me well know that such physical expressions of affection are not something I embrace, if you'll forgive the pun. I'm not a touchy-feely guy. But I was certainly willing to make an exception in Birsha's case.

There were other stories told by Nepalese survivors that day, but these were the ones that stuck in my mind afterward. I returned to my hotel that evening feeling much more fulfilled than I had the previous day.

While I didn't have a specific goal in mind other than to help however possible, I felt that I managed in that regard and did fulfill a "mission." The words of the security agent who had wished me well as I left to fly to Nepal the previous Sunday reemerged in my mind.

My more personal goal was to make it home for Shabbat (and avoid another earthquake while on the runway). So, on a Thursday afternoon, my fourth day in Nepal, I returned to my hotel one last time to gather my belongings and check out.

When I arrived, I noticed that hundreds of tents had been set up on the lawn outside the hotel. A strong sense of guilt shot through me. While I'd been staying in a 5-star hotel (although it was far below that in actual standards), thousands were living in tents not one hundred meters away.

After I'd first arrived in Nepal, someone had asked me what I thought of the people I'd met there. At that time, I mentioned that I was struck by their stoicism. I had also noticed that, when given assistance, many seemed passive — not ungrateful, but almost indifferent. As I talked to survivors more, I realized that gratitude was indeed present and that the seeming stoicism I saw was both a part of their culture and an aftershock of the uncertainty and fear that threatened to overwhelm them.

Still yearning to talk with more survivors, I had the taxi stop and I got out before reaching the hotel entrance. Having given away everything that I'd brought with me, I had nothing of any material worth left to hand. But I wanted to let at least a few more people know that one more person in this world cared about them. In return, I heard personal stories that increased my knowledge and understanding of their situation.

When I approached Yash, I asked him what he was doing to cope with the situation. He teared up, as he stated that it had been almost three weeks, and he still didn't know what would happen. This week's quake made him realize there would likely be more. He asked me to look around, which I did.

People had hardly anything to eat and no access to money, as the banks were all closed. Their homes were destroyed, so they were here on a lawn, unsure what to do or where to go, and it had taken them two weeks to make it this far. He told me that he had lost all the documentation showing the land he owned, so now he was not even sure how he could prove his ownership. If unable to do so, he worried about how he'd make a living.

Narmaya came from a small village near Pokhara. Her English was fluent, so she was able to tell me an amazing story — or rather, miracle — of how she survived the April 25th quake. While her husband was in another village nearby, ironically building a home, she was outside the house, getting ready to wash clothes. Her four-month-old daughter was napping in her crib inside the house. As Narmaya prepared to turn the water on, she felt as though the earth was moving. She attempted to grab the water pipe but fell.

Narmaya turned toward her house and saw it literally collapse before her eyes. She feared that her infant daughter was dead, but her 13-year-old son dug through the rubble and, after four hours, managed to pull out the infant alive. Her baby, Shristi, lay in her arms as she told me this amazing story. Narmaya believed that what had happened was a miracle from G-d, but she was heartbroken that so many others from her village had been killed.

Sudip told me that he was most grateful, as he had his entire family with him in Kathmandu, including his wife, three children, two brothers and their families, his parents, and his wife's parents. While all his clothing, documents, valuables, and land were buried, he said that he had what he valued most. Sudip said that, for the first week after the quake, they slept under corrugated aluminum. By Sunday, they had made their way on foot to Kathmandu, where they slept under the trees and miraculously survived Tuesday's tremors. Again, he stressed that his family members had each other, and they were determined to survive. Sudip's message was inspiring. His positive attitude was one I had seldom seen there.

As the wheels of my plane lifted from the ground on Thursday evening, I had a feeling in my stomach that I'd had nearly twenty-nine years before, when Carol and I had left the Soviet Union after engaging in our undercover Zionist work, passing out Judaica to Soviet refuseniks. It was a feeling of relief that we'd gotten out safely. I vividly remember praying then that the people we met would one day return home.

Friday, I was back home again: to Zion, to Israel. I returned to my children — able to visit with my son for the first time in a while, as he'd been serving in the Israeli Air Force. The following Shabbat, I prayed that the people I'd met would be able to return to a new and safe home. I continue to pray that the citizens of Nepal — every one, individually and communally — garner the strength to overcome the fear that has overtaken them and that they will have the ability, with help from the outside world and the One above, to rebuild a better and stronger nation.

May we all have the fortune to gain happiness, live in peace at home, and learn from one another. The people that I met that week instilled in me a sense of greater pride for who I can be. I hope, I feel, that this experience has made me a better person.

I hope that I represented my country well and will strive to continue to do so on each journey through my life, both locally and abroad. I hope to be able to continue to help others – in Nepal and elsewhere, and I encourage any sympathetic soul to do the same.

While I am certainly not an expert, I do have a keen interest and some experience of working with others on humanitarian aid in countries ranging from the Philippines to the former Soviet Union. Combined with my recent experiences in Nepal, I feel that this gives me some perspective on what the average citizen can do to help out.

For most potential volunteers, a "boots on the ground" approach to assisting, as I did in Nepal, is not advised. There are organized, experienced groups working to provide aid, and in most cases, they need financial support more than anything. In Nepal, I found that what was valued most, other than material assistance, was logistical support.

One should think twice before heading out to help with disaster relief, unless you have relief experience and a specific skill set that is in short supply, for instance, medical aid. While good-hearted people are desperate to help out, an influx of well-meaning but inexperienced individuals is more likely to hinder than help relief efforts. You have to situate yourself in a disaster area in such a way that no one there has to divert energies and resources away from the locals in need in order to take care of you, the well-meaning volunteer. So if you're up for putting your boots on the ground, you should either be experienced and have a plan to be independent or sign up through a reputable relief organization before you head out. Otherwise, the most valuable contribution you can make, other than your prayers, is financial.

I am not going to endorse or discredit any particular fund-raising efforts, but I do caution potential volunteers and donors to check out just where their donation is going before they sign a check. The amount of one's donation that goes directly to relief efforts can vary widely by organization. I've even heard of cases where as little as 10% goes to direct relief. While I was visiting one of the villages in Nepal, I heard from someone who works for a particular organization that is collecting money, which I won't name. He said that while funds may be collected on his behalf, he doubts that he will see much, if any, of the money applied to his actual relief work. In essence, he is being used as a "poster boy" for the fund-raising campaign. That troubles me. So check on the humanitarian organizations before you send them a check.

I have embarked on a project, along with some like-minded souls, to provide housing and/or housing assistance to families that were affected by the earthquakes. 100% of all money raised was given directly to those who were affected. We ended up with around $25,000, which we sent to a village to help them build some prefabricated houses that are designed to withstand earthquakes.

Volunteer work gives me a purpose in life. Nothing gives me greater pleasure than paying it forward. For me, it's a form of therapy. Travel therapy does indeed work. But it's easier for me to fly around the planet, helping strangers, and doing so with compulsive regularity, than to stay at home and work on myself. Sometimes the most difficult, exhausting journey, the one you put off, is the journey within.

Chapter 15

In Search of the Happiest Place on Earth

Bhutan

You will never be happier than you expect. To change your happiness, change your expectations.

— Bette Davis

My travels, aside from the volunteer work projects, have certainly had a *fil rouge* in that I've always been kosher and had to seek out kosher-friendly options in countries unused to providing them. This is part of my interest in Judaism and how it is practiced the world over. It might not seem of such interest in places like England or France, where there is a long, vibrant, and prominent tradition of Judaism, even if it represents a minority. But what about in places like Suriname or Ghana?

Since my diagnosis of living with depression, another through-line has risen among my interests: what makes people in different countries happy, and which countries self-identify as "happiest?"

These are two separate questions, with an added asterisk. Question One: what makes people happy, and does it differ from country to country?

Question Two: which countries self-proclaim as having a happy population? The asterisk? What goes into the self-proclamation? If a government official is leaning over your shoulder as you fill in a form volunteering that you are very happy in that country, then it might not be the most honest of answers.

Question One is more philosophical, but there are some basic ways to approach this. Though I'm Jewish, the answer that I consider best sounds Buddhist: a lack of want. That double-negative means that happy people, or at least content people (we'll get back to the distinction), are those who have what they need — and don't feel a strong urge for more.

Consider the United States. This is a country that I've come to know both as a citizen and resident, but also as a foreign expat, depending on how I would categorize myself. I know it inside and out, quite literally. What I've come to see is that it is a country with an atmosphere, a cultural oxygen, that is highly capitalistic and conspicuous consumption-based. From ads to social media, the message that thrums throughout the country highlights what others have and what you should want to have. This could be material goods (brand-name clothing, snazzy cars, big houses) or a vibe of success and out-and-out happiness. Happiness is potentially problematic, because how many people do you know who are consistently happy? Happy implies a level of euphoria that, to me, seems too much to ask for. It's periodic, the moments of great joy (a professional success, the birth of a child, a warm evening by the fire in a snowstorm, laughing at a favorite film) are brief delights, after which you slot back into your average state. When you live with depression, that average state is far lower than anyone would want, so a moment of happiness might simply mean not feeling bad for an hour, if the other twenty-three hours of that day were marked by doldrums. If your average is, well, average — you feel fine, nothing is missing, you have enough to eat, you're not worried about paying the bills, and so on — then happiness is when something happens that raises you above that middle line.

If we are to fall into the trap of thinking that social media feeds are actually representative of what people's lives are like, then it would appear that everyone is happy and successful most of the time. We naturally compare this to our own state of mind, outside of the curated realm of social media, and this can make us feel bad about ourselves. "I'm not happy and successful the way *everyone* online seems to be, therefore there's something wrong with me." But of course, logically, we know that social media is a highly curated caricature of real life. It is a platform for advertising, both literally ("buy this, lose weight, become a millionaire with my twelve-step program") and metaphorically, with people promoting themselves to the world, sometimes in search of employment, sometimes in the hunt for "likes." One of the worst things someone feeling down can do is browse social media, as it creates a false impression that everyone else is giddy with euphoric success. They aren't.

America in particular is a culture in which one almost feels obliged to broadcast one's happiness. It's even down to greetings in passing on the street. "What's up?" or "How's it going?" are common replacements for "Hello," but no one, aside from your good friends, actually wants to hear your answer. It would be socially odd if you were to reply to such a greeting with anything other than "Great" or "Super." "Actually, I'm not feeling so well today," would confuse your interlocutor. That's not part of the rules of social interaction.

Other countries I've experienced are far slower to introduce America's overt, sometimes in-your-face friendliness and alpha personality. Consider personal photography in Russia. While Americans posing for photographs smile broadly ("Say cheese!") regardless of their mood, Russians generally pose with a straight face. Why smile artificially?

Every year, the UN Sustainable Development Solutions Network surveys people in 150 countries and publishes the World Happiness Report. This is the answer to Question Two. I would rewrite the question, as many people have forgotten it already. One of the report's editors stated, "The big surprise was that, globally, in an uncoordinated way, there have been very large increases in all three forms of benevolence that are asked about in the Gallup World Poll." Part of the poll is to check in on "benevolence," which is associated with a happy population. The three touchstones are whether the population donates to charity, volunteers, or helps strangers.

This is an interesting trifecta to consider. Unhappy people, the thought seems to go, are unlikely to volunteer benevolent acts to help others. I'm not sure that part is true. A good, compassionate, warm-hearted person could feel unhappy but still feel like helping others. I live with depression, but I do all three. Yet some sociologists decided that this was a good measure of happiness.

What is an optimistic sign is that those polled practiced all three benevolent acts 25% more in 2021 than they did before the pandemic. If there were any benefits from it, perhaps they include a feeling of solidarity and a wish to support others in times of need.

The list is also interesting. For the last five years, Finland (perhaps aided by its four-day workweek) has polled as the happiest country on Earth. All the Scandinavian countries are at the top of the list (Denmark is second, Iceland third, Sweden is seventh, Norway eighth). But the attributes that make them such are more about "high quality of life" than "happiness" per se. GDP per capita, healthy life expectancy, low levels of corruption, social support for those in need, high levels of social trust, freedom to make life decisions, and communities in which people look after one another. That all sounds great and important, but it's really about countries that people would want to live in, rather than the happiness of individuals within them. Some of the seemingly happiest, most giving people I've ever met lived in impoverished circumstances.

Here comes the asterisk. The list features exclusively affluent countries in the top ten, with Switzerland fourth, the Netherlands fifth, little Luxembourg sixth, Israel ninth, and New Zealand tenth. With a population that feels that it earns enough and is cared for by its government, then "happiness" seems relatively well-assured (at least for the members of that population who are within the middle-class socioeconomic range — you wonder how broad a socioeconomic swath was polled). It's hard to imagine the American (number sixteen) mentality self-proclaiming as anything other than alpha "winners" in the game of life, whatever the real feelings might be. I think we need separate polls, if we need such polls at all. One list for countries with the highest quality of life, another one about individuals and how content they feel.

In my travels, I've been struck by the warmth, generosity, and apparent happiness of people I've met in countries that check few to none of the quality-of-life boxes in the UN index. Rwanda, for instance, which most people, unfortunately, know only through the issues of ethnic fighting and genocides.

I've loved my travels in Africa, but partly for a selfless/selfish reason: there's so much good you can do there. I associate feeling good about myself with helping those in need. And any help you offer in most African countries is welcome and needed.

I wanted to visit Rwanda because I am intrigued and horrified by the genocides and felt a kinship among peoples who have been victims of genocide. Whether Jews or Armenians, Kurds or Cambodians, or Rwandans, there's a solidarity in collective suffering. When I landed in Rwanda, I flagged a taxi and asked the driver to take me to the Genocide Museum. We did go there, but again, that's the macroscopic, curated view. I also wanted to zoom in and speak to people who are unlikely to be asked by a sympathetic foreigner who's not just a journalist after a headline. So I asked the driver to take me to some villages to meet families who had been damaged by the genocide.

Luckily, I had a friendly driver, but the families were confused. I spent a lot of time walking and chatting with people. Most didn't understand me, linguistically, but in many cases, we managed to build trust. It often went like this: I asked if there was anything I could buy as a gift for the family at a store. "What's the catch?" they would reply. I would convey that there was none. If they wished, I'd like to hear their family story, but no pressure.

Initially, people thought I was a reporter, and so they were suspicious of this foreigner asking questions. But those who chose to speak with me were forthcoming and seemed to appreciate being asked by someone from elsewhere who had no agenda but to listen. Most countries do not have a tradition of counseling or see it as a taboo and don't want to admit going to a counselor. But my sense is that talking through a trauma is something that we humans find helpful. Non-condescending sympathy, or even just a willing ear, can go a long way. Rwanda is a country of millions made orphans by the genocide. Burying hurt within can cause all sorts of problems. A simple chat, even through a language barrier, can provide a salve, releasing the pressure of pent-up anguish.

The Israeli flags I've gotten in the habit of always carrying with me, since the KGB-infiltration days of mine and Carol's youth, came in handy in Rwanda. I was waiting in the hotel lobby to be picked up for a meeting I'd arranged. A local began chatting with me and asked me where I was from.

"Israel," I replied.

He proceeded to quote the Bible far better than I could. "I love the Jewish people," he continued. "I love Israelis. I want to go to Israel. I dream about it. I drew a flag and I have it next to my bed."

"Would you like to have a real Israeli flag?" I asked, somewhat astounded, not only at this interaction, but at the fact that this was finally a moment when my habit of carrying numerous Israeli flags with me to distribute had suddenly found an ideal recipient.

"Oh my," he replied. "Can you send me one?"

"Hold on, I have one in my room." So up I ran and brought it to him. It seemed to be a genuine epiphanic moment for him. And I felt so good about it. He would later send me photos of the flag displayed in his home.

It has been in places like Rwanda that I've met people who seem more open, generous, welcoming, and hospitable than in many of the "first world" countries I've visited. Maybe there's more to benevolence than being in a socioeconomic position to offer help to others.

Uganda was another place where I had a similarly positive experience and this time when visiting an ancient Jewish group there. Back in 1903, Uganda was proposed as an alternative site for a Jewish state, when Palestine was considered too complicated a location. The British colonial secretary at the time, Joseph Chamberlain, offered a 5,000 square mile (13,000 square kilometer) territory on the Mau Plateau (today this is a part of Kenya). The World Zionist Organization described Uganda as an "antechamber to the Holy Land." A strong and ancient Jewish population has always been present in Ethiopia, and so there is a historical rationale for this. The Russian Jews of the World Zionist Organization were incensed by this counteroffer, feeling that Palestine should be the only option. They stormed out of the conference. But the idea was put to a vote and the plan was passed, 295 votes to 177. For three years, a delegation considered the suggestion. But a number of factors led to them politely declining the offer. The land was considered wild and dangerous, and the major population of Maasai there did not take kindly to the idea of being displaced.

Yet, a Jewish local community established itself there. The Abayudaya people, based in and around the town of Mbale, in today's eastern Uganda, number just a few thousand, but they have been observant, practicing Jews since precisely 1919, keeping kosher and observing Shabbat. Most are Reform or Conservative, but a community called the Putti converted to Orthodox Judaism in 2016.

Why so specific a date for the origins of Judaism there? The story goes that a military leader of the Muganda people (which represents around 15% of the Ugandan population) called Semei Kakungulu was first converted to Christianity by British missionaries when Uganda was a British territory. The deal was that, if Kakungulu became Christian, the British would provide support for him and make him king. But they never followed through on their half of the deal, even shrinking his territory. In 1913 Kakungulu joined a sect called the Bamalaki, which adhered to a hybrid belief system that incorporated elements of Christianity and Judaism, with their own interpretative twist (for example, they refused vaccinations and western medicine, based on their interpretation of the Old Testament as forbidding it). Kakungulu was an avid member and student of the Old Testament. He introduced circumcision of males as a practice, but the Bamalaki didn't like this idea, not wishing to be Jews per se, just borrowing elements of Judaism that suited them. Kakungulu was said to have replied to this by stating "Then I am a Jew." His conviction was strengthened by the arrival of a foreign Jew in 1920 known as Yosef. Yosef introduced Ashkenazi Jewish practices while living with the community for half a year. Kakungulu volunteered to be circumcised, along with his sons, and declared that he and the community he led were Jewish. This community of his followers and their descendants, though small in number, have practiced Judaism ever since.

I'd heard about the Jews of Uganda and was curious to visit the country. One of the through-lines of my travels has been getting to know Jewish communities living in countries in which one might be surprised to find any more than a smattering of Jews.

Uganda doubly intrigued me because I've long admired Yoni Netanyahu (he happens to be the brother of Israeli prime minister, Benjamin Netanyahu, but that's neither here nor there).

Yoni is a hero of mine for his role in the 1976 Operation Entebbe. On June 27, 1976, an Air France Airbus setting out from Tel Aviv and bound for Paris, with 248 passengers, was hijacked by two members of the Popular Front for the Liberation of Palestine and two Germans. The hijackers demanded the release of forty Palestinians imprisoned in Israel as well as thirteen prisoners held elsewhere. The plane was diverted and ended up in Uganda's main airport. There the hijackers separated the Israeli hostages from the non-Israelis. The non-Israelis were all released and flown to Paris. Ninety-four Israeli passengers, and the twelve airline crew members, remained as hostages. They would be killed, the hijackers said, if their prison release request was not fulfilled.

Yoni led a commando unit that rescued Israeli hostages being held at Entebbe Airport in Uganda. All of the hostage takers were killed, as well as four of the hostages: 102 of the 106 hostages were rescued. But Yoni was killed in action — the only member of the rescue team to lose his life. Yoni was an Israeli superhero and a martyr. Uganda was the place of pilgrimage to pay homage to his heroism.

So along came another foreign Jew to Uganda, Stuart by name, to visit the Abayudaya.

I flew into Entebbe Airport and set off for this Jewish community, which consists of eight rural villages. I traveled with seven suitcases full of Judaica, including the Israeli flags I always bring abroad. I was greeted warmly — they weren't used to visitors. I immediately recognized that they were Jews. Each of the eight villages had its own synagogue and each had slight variations on their practices and beliefs, none of them entirely agreeing.

I spent several days visiting all the villages. There were some 500 schoolchildren who were particularly delighted with the flags I'd brought. They couldn't have been more welcoming. At one point I really had to use the restroom, but I didn't know the proper etiquette. Should I gingerly sneak behind a tree? There were no bathrooms in sight. I asked someone where to go, thinking I'd be directed to a secluded shrub or something. Instead, I was escorted out of the village. Way out of the village. A two-kilometer walk out of the village in fact. Good thing I didn't have to go too badly.

We came upon what looked like a well, but it was in fact four low walls surrounding a hole in the ground. This was the guest restroom.

While my visits to Rwanda and Uganda filled me with a sense of warmth, neither place has a reputation for happiness. Rwanda, in particular, has just about the saddest recent history of any nation on Earth. I've visited so many localities of sadness that my thoughts turned to visiting a place renowned for its happiness.

Bhutan is often mentioned as "the happiest country in the world." But according to the UN report, it's the 95th happiest country in the world. The problem with the report is that it focuses on socioeconomics and government policy. It doesn't cover how inclusive social groups are, population health in general (just life expectancy), national suicide levels (Bhutan has 5.1 per 100,000 people, while Finland has 13.4), how frequently people laugh and smile, how much people enjoy their lives, how often people feel anxious or depressed. These are far more difficult measures to take, but they seem to me better indicators of contentment. Maybe we need two separate lists: one is for countries with a high quality of life, places you might like to live if you're flexible enough to choose; and a separate list looking at the actual "happiness" of the people. The UN introduced the Human Development Index in 2017, which covers more bases (education rates for children up to age fifteen, sanitation, clean drinking water access), but it still looks macroscopically, rather than at individuals.

The Bhutan government introduced a "Gross National Happiness" score, which provides questionnaires for 15,000 residents of various countries. Bhutan scored highest. Some economic theorists, like Richard Easterlin of the University of Southern California, have advocated for a happiness-based economic model rather than the finance-centered one that is most used today.

When I learned about Bhutan's Gross National Happiness system, I wanted to travel there to check it out. While there I met a lot of people to talk about what makes for a happy population. I spoke to some psychiatrists, gurus, government officials, and just folks I met out and about there. There's a minimal recorded suicide rate, which sounds good on paper but doesn't necessarily mean anything. You've got the word "recorded" in there, which means an official has to decide to list an incident, and there's nothing about attempts. Of note is that there are lots of dogs — everyone loves dogs — and no stoplights. I'm not sure I have anything against stoplights, but there you go. The lack of stoplights doesn't seem to negatively affect traffic. The king there is highly respected in a way that came across to me as genuine. He travels extensively, visiting villages, really integrating with his people. So a benevolent monarch seems like a good thing.

What came across in all my conversations was a lack of external pressure. Most individuals do not feel pressured — whether from the government or your boss or your peers and neighbors. You are what you are, and that's good enough. So that's a nice definition of happiness: a lack of external pressures.

Part of this may be down to Bhutan being a primarily Buddhist country. The Buddhist ethos of desire being the root of evil — I think there's something to that. Wanting what you don't have is a form of unhappiness. Of course, you need to have your basics covered. If you want food and don't have it that's got nothing to do with a survey of happiness. But wanting material goods, wanting what others have, feeling like you lack while others thrive — that certainly can lead to anxiety and stress. Is a lack of desire synonymous with happiness? Again, I think it leads more to a condition of contentment. Happiness proper remains an outlier human emotion, one to be cherished when it occurs, but to proactively seek it out can lead to unhappiness, and stress at not feeling happy (when it feels like you should, and others do).

I've come to think that a better rating would be "the most content countries" rather than "the happiest." I'm not sure I trust "happy." There's subconscious pressure to self-describe as "happy" when that's really an outlier state for us humans. Contentment, on the other hand, feels more honest. A lack of want, having your basic needs met plus a little more to cover modest additions, seems like what we should be aiming for. Believe me, when feeling depressed, contentment seems enough of a goal. Happiness, the high point of the sine wave, feels frustratingly distant and almost inappropriate to aim for. When it comes, we can be grateful for it. But it's an exercise in further frustration to seek it.

My journey has been much more modest in its aspiration. Rather than seeking happiness, I've sought *not* feeling awful. That's a big difference. And I've made quite a study out of both why I, and so many people around the world, feel this way, and what methods are available to try to pull us all from the brink of hopelessness to a state of okay-ness. Because that okay-ness can feel a million miles away.

Chapter 16

The Me Project:
Investing in My Own Mental Health

Stuart's Right Frontal Cortex

To love oneself is the beginning of a lifelong romance.

— Oscar Wilde

I first went to a therapist in 2008 and was with him for about a year. This was when my grandfather died and the Israir troubles took place, so I felt I needed help primarily with those two external factors. I was not in a great place, and I think it helped — we had a great dynamic. I only stopped when we moved to Israel. I would resume during the pandemic, in the summer of 2021.

Here's the thing with therapy. There are many schools of thought, approaches, training methods to choose from, and they are more developed all the time. You want to work with a therapist with whom you feel comfortable, but that's just part of it. You also want to be on the cutting edge if the traditional approaches haven't helped as much as you'd like. If your situation is such that you'd benefit from medication, then you'll need a psychiatrist —

those are the only therapists who can prescribe medication. Some might like the Freudian psychoanalysis approach, in which the doctor sits out of the patient's line of vision, the patient is on a couch or divan and the doctor tries to coax tucked-away, subconscious memories through dialogue. That is a very slow, long-term therapy approach.

In stark contrast stands cognitive behavioral therapy, which might only require a few sessions to sort out an issue. This approach tends to work best when there's a specific trigger for anxiety, like a phobia. For example, if you're afraid of spiders.

One method is to "flood" thinking about the thing that worries you so much that your mind grows used to it, even bored of it, and it no longer triggers an upsetting response. This is a component of CBT called "exposure therapy." The therapist helps you envision a scenario involving spiders that would normally upset you, and which your mind wants to avoid. Sometimes this is scripted, and you read it, or you can record yourself narrating the sequence so that each time you "flood" you are getting the same story and sequence of images that accompany it. As you go about your day, your mischievous mind wants to bring the frightening or upsetting idea to the fore. Each time it does so, you deflect it, saying to yourself, "No, not now. I'll give you worry-time later." Worry-time is a set amount of time, for instance fifteen minutes a day, during which you will flood and devote a block of focused time to what worries you. You can trick your mind into holding off on introducing that worry regularly throughout your day if you give your mind a block of time later to scratch the proverbial itch and worry about it then. During worry-time each day, you flood about the issue, doing it so often and so repetitively that your mind eventually shrugs its shoulders and says the equivalent of "what's the big deal." The thing that worried you has been rendered mundane and impotent because you've overplayed the scenario. The benefit of this flooding and worry-time system is that it gives you homework so you can feel proactive. The more time you flood in confined worry-time blocks, the sooner you'll feel better. The therapist is there to help you through the process but you're doing almost all the work on your own time. For this reason, sometimes a few sessions are all you need.

Another cognitive-behavioral approach is to incrementally expose yourself to what you fear. You might begin by just thinking about a spider. Then you move on to looking at a cartoonish drawing of a spider. Then a photograph of a spider. Then you watch a nature documentary about spiders. Then you finally go to the insect section of your local zoo, with your therapist, and see spiders in person. Each encounter, however far removed (even if just looking at a drawing of a spider), feels like a tiny triumph, a moment of empowerment. On you go, until you can see a spider in person and not have the clutch of fear seize you.

These approaches treat symptoms without bothering with the underlying issue. Sometimes that's enough. You might not need to unearth the long-buried formative trauma of when your 11-year-old cousin Larry thought it would be funny to throw a toy rubber spider into your crib and, from that moment on, you've always been terrified of spiders. You just want that seizure of fear when you see one to go away.

I didn't have a specific anxiety trigger that I could point to. And, as I'm learning, does it really matter? I didn't know which therapeutic approach would work best for me. I knew I preferred not to take a pharmaceutical approach (they work well for many, it just didn't feel right for me), but that was about it. Some might argue that it's best to try one approach at a time, so you know which one is working for you. If you have tummy troubles then you might give up gluten or lactose or meat — or you might give up all three at once and, as long as you're feeling better, not worry about which one was causing the indigestion. That's the angle I took. I want to try as much as possible as quickly as possible, to feel better sooner. I'm still not bothered to know which approach helps most. As long as I'm feeling better — or rather, not so much worse that I am no longer with you — then that qualifies as a success. I do recognize and try to share with others that caring for your mental health is a lifelong process. There's no get-better-quick approach. I've tried them, and they just don't work. It requires a lifestyle change, and that change begins with acceptance.

Part of depression is shifting your expectations to more modest, miniature positives. "I'm still alive today," may not sound like much of a victory, but it sure feels like one. If you can see a single thing to look forward to in your day — a cup of tea, a TV show, a warm fire in the hearth, a hug (and I've never liked to hug, so maybe I should try it) — then that's a step in the right direction, as those of us with depression can feel like there's *nothing* to look forward to, nothing to live for.

Modalities of therapy are generally directed at treating symptoms of a trauma that cause anxiety and/or identifying the root cause and, by expressing and exploring it, uprooting it altogether. Cognitive-behavioral is symptom-focused. Psychoanalysis is root cause focused. The two can work well together, but therapists usually specialize in one or the other. Hence my "more is more" approach to getting help.

There are those of us with genetic predispositions to mental health issues. It demonstrably runs in families. But an estimated 70% of adults in the United States report having experienced at least one significant trauma in their lives (and that doesn't take into account those who had a formative trauma but aren't aware of it). Of those, some 6% develop post-traumatic stress disorder (PTSD). We think of PTSD as something that affects soldiers, and it certainly can. Being in battle and seeing comrades killed is a very obvious form of trauma. But PTSD can be far more subtle. It's stress, anxiety, depression, insomnia, suicidal thoughts that negatively impact your life, the origins of which are from a trauma that may have happened years, even decades ago, and which you may not consciously recall. I do not have a single formative trauma of which I'm aware. That doesn't mean there isn't one. Concern for Dafna and the issues with Israir could qualify, but my sense is that I've been depressed since long before either of those moments.

There are numerous therapies that help with PTSD.

Prolonged exposure therapy is the gradual exposure to a spider I mentioned above. Incremental exposure in a controlled way that lessens the upset.

Cognitive processing therapy involves a therapist challenging the unhelpful beliefs surrounding events. For example, maybe a soldier feels like it was his "fault" that a comrade was killed, when in fact there was nothing he could have done and his actions actually saved others.

There are some more exotic-sounding approaches, like EMDR, or Eye Movement Desensitization and Reprocessing. It's exotic because it's not a talking therapy, but rather a series of exercises. The doctor asks you to recount or focus on aspects of your traumatic event while your eyes are focused on her moving hand, causing your eyes to dart from side to side, engaging both sides of the brain — a process called bilateral stimulation. Developed by Dr. Francine Shapiro in 1987, a 2014 study found that 80-90% of patients using this therapy felt relief from their trauma within three sessions. That sounds promising, but it's most helpful when there was a single event trauma — say, a car accident — and you know exactly what the trauma was.

I tried cranial-sacral therapy, an alternative approach that involves gentle palpitation of the cranium — a light head massage, in other words. It's a therapy that has not been proven effective in extensive tests, but which many feel helped them. It's one of those things that doesn't hurt to try. I tried massage therapy, too, which makes the body feel better and, for some, helps the mind as well.

Acceptance and Commitment Therapy (ACT) does not try to "fix" a mental health issue but rather accepts it as simply a part of the human mind. Instead of trying to repel the bad feeling, like an invisible tumor that must be extracted and destroyed, lest it destroy you, this approach teaches how to live with the issue, working around it, without the goal of being rid of it indefinitely.

The idea that we are in some sort of wrestling match with our own mind is, well, mind-bending. If I think to myself, "Brain, stop trying to mess with me," then surely it is my own brain telling my brain to stop mucking around. How does that work? Some describe an instinctual "reptilian brain" as one that is reactive, trying to be helpful but often causing problems due to its primal reactions. Being afraid of spiders might have helped our ancestors but today most of us live far from any spider that could harm us. This is contrasted with the "monkey brain" as it is sometimes called, which is more logical, empathetic, reflective, understanding, and problem-solving. So in this analogy, the monkey brain is telling the lizard brain to stop messing about, though, in fact, both are part of Stuart's mind. Confusing stuff.

Internal Family Systems Therapy expands on this idea to imagine an Inner Self that is compassionate and loving and can help heal mental and emotional wounds by helping us better understand our relationships. By imagining this Inner Self as a benevolent, helpful aspect of our minds, this approach uses mindfulness and acceptance to stimulate self-compassion.

The list goes on: hypnotherapy, somatic therapy, psychodynamic, accelerated resolution, narrative, inner child, trauma systems, even art and music therapies, where engaging in the arts acts as both an emotional release and a portal of inquiry for your therapist, who can analyze the art you create for what subconscious issues it might hint at. Maybe dolphin therapy — engaging with animals — would do the trick? I did cuddle a panda for thirty seconds once.

TRAVEL THERAPY

Each of these approaches has helped many. By which I mean, there are many people suffering from trauma, anxiety, and depression who report having been helped by all of the therapies I listed here, and many that I haven't. Some are more scientifically proven than others, but I don't care. I'll try anything that might work and that won't make matters worse.

I've been a good student of all this. I read books. Lots of them. By Bessel van der Kolk, a Dutch therapist best known for the best-selling book *The Body Keeps the Score,* and president of the International Society for Traumatic Stress Studies. By Janina Fisher from Harvard Medical School, who writes on the legacy of trauma, as in *Healing the Fragmented Selves of Trauma Survivors: Overcoming Self-Alienation.* By Pat Ogden, author of *Trauma and the Body.* These three therapists are also linked, collaborating with one another. So if there's a "school of thought" that I've focused on, it is theirs. Most of my therapists studied under them.

Here's the thing about therapies. I'm a tremendous believer in them, but I'm not sure I'm a believer in one specific modality over another. I think all have different skills and it's important to learn them and use them as needed. I'm a big believer and follower of the integrated approach.

But what's really proven best for me is *Travel Therapy*.

Chapter 17

Addicted to Helping Others: Travels to Aid Refugees

Greece

If we all did the things we are capable of doing, we would literally astound ourselves.

— Thomas Edison

Part of that travel therapy is my travel to help strangers. I'm of no importance to anyone outside of my immediate family. But perhaps I can help beyond those confines by offering my energies to those in need. And by telling their stories.

One of the ways I have learned to get a sense of self-worth, to self-care, to raise my self-esteem is in volunteer service to those in need throughout the world. As you've seen, I have found myself at the site of recent earthquakes, tidal waves, winter storms, and war-torn zones. Rarely have I felt more challenged than during a series of trips to volunteer in Greece.

In 2015, the world was inundated with news and stories of the Syrian refugee crisis. Hearing all this, each of us was challenged with the difficult question: Where do I stand?

It's important that people recognize that every family history includes ancestors who were refugees at one time or another. I don't just mean Jews, who have been subject to forced diasporas and have fled violence over the millennia. Today's generation might not know the story, and even if they did, their predecessors might not have been a refugee in the crisis sense of the word. But no one should feel that refugees are somehow "others," with nothing in common with those of us who are fortunate enough not to be refugees at the moment. Humans have an obligation to help other humans. I can't stand when people react to my desire to help by saying, "You don't owe them anything." I totally disagree with that.

Certainly, no matter where you stand, one thing is true: no one — not one decent person — wants to see innocent victims of violence and oppression suffer or starve or die. The Syrian refugees have already survived war and poverty. They have crossed deserts, mountains, and rough seas. Many of those who survived now have arrived in Europe with little more than the clothes they wear.

Since this crisis hit the headlines, I've felt completely consumed with sadness, guilt, and helplessness over the humanitarian crisis caused by the refugee exodus. My people have been strangers in a strange land, but they left en masse, whereas the refugees of this era fled piecemeal, not as a collective but each family grasping desperately for a foothold beyond their blasted homeland. I honestly was unable to think of anything else since that wave of refugees surged across the news and social media platforms.

But aside from the obvious activity of donating money, what can people like us do to help those who are suffering? I'm not the sort to jump headlong into something. I brooded and wondered and worried for six months. I wanted to do something, but I wasn't sure what. I wanted to feel that I could have some clear impact, however small, on even one person. But how?

At the same time, I was curious, intrigued, fascinated to learn more. To find out the truth behind the so-called "refugee problem." Knowing how the news media reports events, with so much experience of my eye on "war-torn Israel," my cynicism is understandable, wondering whether the truth about what was happening a few hundred kilometers away from me was accurately reflected in media portrayals. I wanted to experience the reality of the situation, unfiltered by any media bias or hyperbole.

A trip to Damascus or Aleppo was out of the question. It was a war zone, and American Israeli Jews were the people least advised to go anywhere near Syria. So where could I find the truth? How to separate the truth from the shrapnel of lies, misinformation, and incomplete outtakes found on Facebook or Twitter? There are multiple sides to every story, and those sides can be difficult to discern. I was eager to see the situation for myself — to help satisfy my own curiosity and to guide me in determining how I could help.

I learned that there was a severe shortage of volunteers in Greece. That felt like the answer, at least to the question "Where?" I decided to spend a week in Athens, helping where I could. For me, solutions to life's problems, whether my own or those of others, come through travel. Some folks stay home to sort themselves out, or to lend a hand. I need to move. I needed a destination for that key chapter. It was Greece.

According to the International Rescue Committee and others I spoke with when I was in Athens, approximately 2,000 refugees were arriving daily on Greece's shores. The majority of these individuals and families are fleeing the brutal civil war in Syria, which had raged for five years by the time I arrived.

The International Organization for Migration at the time estimated that more than a million migrants and refugees had found their way to Europe over the course of 2016. This represented the largest mass migration since the end of World War II. The route for most of these individuals was by way of the eastern Aegean Sea, crossing over from Turkey to outlying Greek islands such as Chios, Kos, and Lesbos. In 2015, approximately 810,000 migrants and refugees arrived in Greece from the countries of Syria and neighboring Iraq and Afghanistan. Many arrived in rubber dinghies or less-than-seaworthy boats and over 700 people had lost their lives making that journey by the time I'd arrived.

In addition to the over 800,000 who had arrived in Greece, almost 200,000 had arrived on other European shores: Italy, Spain, Cyprus, and Malta, by the time I was ready to volunteer. Whatever the destination, the numbers represented a quadrupling of European emigres from 2014. The number only ballooned afterward.

As has happened so often in my life, I'll learn about a crisis and a siren rings in my mind, summoning me to drop everything and set off to "save the world." I headed off to Greece on my own, without any organization sponsoring or awaiting me there. That's usually how I approach my volunteer work. I figure that these humanitarian organizations have their hands full enough as it is, and I don't want to be an extra burden. I'm there to relieve the burden. So, I'd just land, show up, and get stuck in, doing whatever I thought needed doing.

I didn't tell my family where I was going. I didn't want them to worry. Again, my role, as I saw it, was to relieve others, and that included not adding the weight of concern to my immediate family members. They thought I was off on a business trip.

I was, sort of. The business of helping. I wouldn't pack heavily, as I preferred to support the local economy. I would bring money with which I would buy supplies and food locally. I'd check in with distribution centers, which were often waiting for shipments and inevitably low on one thing or another. By far the most common need, besides food, were diapers and wet wipes.

My wife knew where I was going and supported me but with a few conditions. I couldn't say I was Jewish. I couldn't say I was from Israel. And I couldn't wear a kippah. The gist was that I had to be religiously incognito. Jews throughout history have been subject to discrimination and worse. Even in my capacity as a volunteer, you just never knew. So it was the path of least resistance to be religion-neutral. I would go as a human hoping to help. No other identifiers were needed.

I agreed with these stipulations. I wasn't going to be seen as a Jewish volunteer. I wasn't going to be seen at all. I was going to help. Period. Carol's list reminded me of my high school days in Yeshiva when we would come to a Bnei Akiva youth program on Shabbat. We'd have to promise the rabbi three things: that we wouldn't talk to girls; that I would pray during the afternoon service; and that I would return right after Shabbat. Back then I secretly thought to myself, *Well, if I cover two out of the three requests, I'm on the right track.* I figured I'd aim for the same batting average in Greece when it came to fulfilling my wife's requirements.

I arrived in Greece with hope, trepidation, and curiosity. I looked forward to interacting with as many people as I could — both to provide support and to be educated by them. In the course of my time there, I learned more than I had ever anticipated.

After my first day, I spent a lot of time following children around, attempting to engage them in conversations through drawings, smiles, and games, though we rarely shared a common language. I also made sure they had plenty to eat. There was food in the relief centers, but I noticed that it took forever to distribute through the normal channels they used. I tried to speed things up by borrowing a few volunteers and heading to a store. I would then bring these foodstuffs to the refugees I'd met. With a couple of other volunteers, I also bought diapers and baby wipes at the local store and brought them back to one of the refugee centers. I kept saying to myself that *all* children — no matter what migration status, origin, or religion — have a right to a safe and happy childhood.

I met many amazing adults as well — individuals who educated me about the refugee situation through both words and deeds. I think of many as true heroes who made difficult choices for the sake of their families and their future.

The first time I had a deeper conversation with an adult, I had a really hard time lying. I had promised to pretend to be someone I wasn't. My "cover story" was that I was not a Jewish volunteer from Israel wishing to help Syrians, but an a-religious volunteer from Johnson City, Tennessee — a location that sounded as un-Jewish as I could think of.

The refugee camp I wound up visiting repeatedly, spending two-to-four days a month there, was just outside of Athens, near the former Olympic Stadium. On my first visit, some of the folks running the refugee camp were showing me around, when a refugee approached and said that he needed slippers. So I went to the depot where donated items were stored and I rummaged around and found him a pair of slippers. All this time we got to talking. He had been injured by the opposition in Syria and there was this miracle — he said, "I was hurt, and I was airlifted ... to Israel." Now, I couldn't say what I wanted to because I'd promised Carol. But I'm sitting there thinking how crazy it is for me to be so guarded, when this Syrian refugee is telling me how great Israel is. And I want to join in and tell him where I'm from, but I can't. I have to be from Johnson City, Tennessee. At that point, I decided that I couldn't do it. I couldn't lie. Because guilt is my co-pilot. He and I spent a few hours talking and it was so meaningful, or rather it became a level more meaningful when I no longer had this gauze of a lie separating us.

That night I emailed my wife (because, well, guilt is my co-pilot) and wrote, "I'm sorry, I can't do this." She was supportive and replied, "It's okay, do what you have to do."

On the following trip to Athens, I met the man who I got closest to through all my volunteer trips — we're in touch to this day. He's an amazing person and was only twenty-three at the time. He was a refugee in the camp, too, but spent his time volunteering to help other refugees, as it helped him deal with his own trauma.

That would become a diagnosis I'd give myself.

We wound up working as volunteers in the same warehouse together. He asked where I was from, and I said that I was from Israel. This surprised him, as we'd been getting along really well. Suddenly he didn't want to have anything to do with me. How absurd, just because of where I'm from, nothing to do with who I am. He kept to his own at the warehouse for a while. It was a big space, and we were constantly on the move — someone would come in and say what they needed, and we'd find a match, and put together orders. We didn't speak the rest of the day, but when our shift ended, I said, "Will you be here tomorrow?"

"Yes," he replied.

"Okay, I'll see you then." And we went our separate ways.

The next day we were back at the warehouse and got to talking again. Slowly. I guess he'd slept on the idea that there was an Israeli volunteering, and he saw that I wasn't a threat. I understood his stance — he'd been living with what he'd been told about Israel, and the national narrative wasn't flattering. Perhaps he'd never met a Jew before. But I didn't fit the profile he'd been taught.

Since he was a refugee, he wasn't allowed to leave the camp. So I began to bring him meals from outside, which he very much appreciated. We started spending time chatting after work hours ended. I'd be there for two or three days a month, and I was scheduled to head home the next day.

"Look, next time I'm back I'd like to bring you a gift," I said. "But I'd rather buy you what you need, what you can really use."

He was taken aback in a good way. He didn't know what to say. He was such a humble guy who'd been through too much pain in his short life to date.

Our budding friendship grew with each of my visits, but it wasn't a good thing that he remained there, month after month, stuck in the camp. He was trying to reach Germany, but he kept being denied permission. My gift to him ended up being a plane ticket to Germany. With a little help, he was finally accepted as an emigree to Germany, but he had no money to buy the ticket.

That was the best ticket I've ever bought.

He's still in Germany today. He deals with a lot of trauma, but he's beginning to talk about it, little by little. It took years for him to really see he could open up to me, particularly about mental health. Opening up wasn't something that was part of his culture, and mental health was taboo. If I've helped him in any way, I'm grateful for that.

So much of refugee coverage is about blindingly large but anonymous numbers (800,000 refugees sounds enormous but it is also purely theoretical — match them all to faces and stories, and it really hits home). So, I vowed to remember the faces and the names and share some of their stories.

Javid. When I first arrived in Athens, I went to the Notara Refugee Solidarity Center. There I met Javid, an Afghani who shared with me that nobody wants to leave his or her country or family. Afghans aren't fleeing by choice or making a reflective decision to come to Europe.

The reasons for Javid's leaving quickly become clear. "The Taliban, for instance, kills its opponents, takes them off buses, cuts their heads off, and leaves them in the streets," he explained to me, using both hands to gesture in a beheading motion. "Winter may slow down the number of Afghans coming to Europe, but if there is war, then people will keep coming."

Javid added that he hopes his family will return home to Afghanistan one day. He sadly shared with me, "We miss our relatives and our home a lot — we never wanted to leave."

Mohsen. Mohsen arrived here from Iran. I met him as I was cleaning out the showers. (As I never do this at home, I can't vouch for the quality of my work.) Mohsen was looking for shower slippers, as he had just arrived in Athens that morning. I asked the person in charge for assistance, and she said that, after lunch, she would attempt to find some for him. I then followed up and learned that they had no slippers left. I was told that Mohsen should just be happy they let him in at all.

Unfortunately, these words demonstrated an attitude that I saw quite a bit with the Greeks in the refugee camps. I want to believe that they were overtired and just had blunt personalities, but even so, I was disturbed. Many of the workers failed to treat their "guests" with dignity or compassion. At times they seemed to treat them more like criminals.

As for Mohsen, he spoke English fairly well — the best I had yet heard from a refugee. We began a question-and-answer session. He asked where I was from, and I told him I was from the USA. At that, he replied, "Oh, Iran and America aren't friends. Iran is friends with everyone except America and Israel." Well, my thought was: *you're probably speaking to the wrong person, then!* But inside I felt a strong urge to help him. Most of all, I wanted to make him smile.

Mohsen and I walked around the nearby soccer field several times. As the conversation warmed, he showed me photos of the 6-month-old daughter he had left behind in Iran with his wife. I asked him about his plans, and he told me he was planning to leave within a couple of days and head north, cross the border, and make his way to Germany. He was just waiting for a German friend to wire him some money.

Mohsen asked me how old I thought he looked. While he looked close to sixty, I was afraid I might insult him, so I said "forty." He replied that this is what happened to him in Iran — that was why he had to get out. He said that everyone in Iran ages quickly because of what's there. He said, "I'm 32."

Then he shared that he doesn't really think that America and Israel are the true enemies. As I made this trip with the notion that I was strictly "from the USA," so as to avoid any unnecessary potential conflict or prejudice against Israel, I agreed with him that I also knew many nice people from Israel and that they contribute so much to the world! He gave a small reaffirming nod.

When a special pass could be arranged, I liked to bring refugees to the store with me and buy whatever they needed for them directly. I couldn't get one for Mohsen, so later, I went to the store and bought Mohsen some slippers and other goods, wishing I could have bought enough for all. I told him I would see him the next day. All night, I thought about him and developed a list of additional questions that I really wanted to ask him the next day.

Unfortunately, I couldn't find Mohsen the next morning. None of the other Iranians seemed to know where he was. I hope and pray that he is safely on his way to Germany and his dreamed-of new life.

Yazen. Yazen is a Yazidi from Sinjar in Iraq. I met him one day while I was preparing breakfast for the guests. He helped me pour milk and line the glasses up on the counters. As we worked, he told me his story, in pretty good English.

Before the terrorists arrived in his city, Yazen worked as a student translator for foreign oil companies. When the terrorists came, they began to kidnap women and children and murdered many people.

"My mother and sister were taken by them," Yazen explained, "And I may never see them again. There is genocide happening there, and people need to know about this!" He emphasized the point, turning to me as if it were solely my duty, "You must tell the people."

And so I do, by sharing Yazen's story and that of many others. I cannot change what has happened to these people, and I am uncertain how much I helped them. But I *can* share their stories.

Yazen and I spoke for a long time. I learned of all his struggles and his journey so far. He even explained Yazidi culture to me, and I really enjoyed listening to him and learning about things I had never experienced. Along with Yazen, every person I met during my week in Greece taught me something in some way.

Shirzad and Novi. Arriving from Kabul, Afghanistan, Shirzad and Novi made the journey with many of their family members. They arrived on the northern shores of Lesbos one morning earlier that month. After an eight-hour walk, they arrived at a registration center outside the Lesbos capital of Mytilene. Shirzad noted that the long walk was made even more difficult by a waterlogged backpack, but he barely noticed the fatigue. To get to this point, the two had already crossed four countries and covered nearly 3,000 miles, mostly on foot. Traveling from Kabul, they passed through Pakistan, crossed into Iran, then traveled into Turkey and across the country's Aegean coast, before they piled into an inflatable rubber boat for the ride to Greece.

During their almost 20-day journey, they were shot at by Iranian border guards, loaded into the back of a pickup truck for a grueling, daylong drive across an Iranian desert, and held for ransom by smugglers who they had thought were assisting them. They were forced by their captors to give up most of the money they had brought with them, but they felt they had no choice in order to stay alive.

When they arrived on Greek shores, Shirzad and Novi joined other migrants and refugees at a café in Lesbos that has become something of an unofficial base for non-Syrian immigrants.

They are part of the changing demographics of European refugees. Earlier that year, Syrians constituted the majority of individuals risking the journey to Europe. However, the makeup of passengers in the inflatable boats reaching the shores of Lesbos changed. Iraqis, Iranians, Afghanis, Moroccans, Somalis, and Bangladeshis were arriving in greater numbers than ever before.

After two weeks in Greece, the pair has almost completely run out of money. While in Lesbos, they bought a tent and set it up at the main port, the parking lot of which was filled with such tents. Garbage was everywhere, dumpsters overflowing. They ended up camping out under one of the café windows while waiting for ferry tickets to Athens. While they waited, the café owner let them charge their phones and use his Wi-Fi. The family was finally able to send them additional money, enabling them to take the ferry to Athens. With funds low but hopes still high, Shirzad and Novi faced an uncertain future as they sought final asylum.

Adnan. Adnan, who arrived here from Syria, introduced himself to me when I was working in the "shoe department" at the port in Piraeus, Greece. He began by showing me the hole in his foot. Admittedly, I was a bit grossed out by the sight (my stomach is not my mightiest organ), but I was certainly inspired to help him find the right shoe to fit his injured foot. Adnan did not speak English, and I do not speak Arabic, so we started off our conversation with hand signals. Luckily, I was able to locate an Arabic-speaking assistant to translate for us.

What Adnan told me gave me chills. He related that he was so happy to be in Greece now and was hoping to leave with his family that night for the northern border. There they would begin a trek across Europe to Sweden, where he had friends. He was understandably concerned about his injured foot, so I went with him to the first aid station, where we secured some cream and the assurance that he would be fine.

Adnan told me of his attack and his surgery. He said that he wished he could go back to the hospital where his surgery was performed after his attack. I asked him where the hospital was, and his answer brought quick tears to my eyes.

He said it was in Israel.

I asked the name of the hospital, and he said, "Ziv." As I hadn't revealed my origins during my times in Greece — and wasn't about to — I just said, "I hear they have excellent doctors there." I found myself feeling so lucky — lucky to be part of a true democracy, and *so* lucky to have the life I have. I hope and pray that Adnan and his family will also find that life in their new land.

So many people, so many stories. They speak to the situation more than any quoting of facts and figures ever could.

There were three recurring thoughts I had, amid all the confusion and emotional challenges.

First, the resonance of history. Not for one second would I compare the conditions and treatment of the refugees to what many of our families endured during the Holocaust, but it made the thought of what they endured even more painful than I had ever thought possible. I have studied and researched much of the Holocaust but learning facts and truly feeling their impact are not the same thing. In World War II, the issue was: Shall we annihilate Jews from the world? Thank G-d history will not allow that to happen to any people of any race or religion. But the Jews of World War II had no place to go, no homeland awaiting them. Those from the war-battered regions of Syria, Iraq, and Afghanistan have somewhere to go, as there are over twenty-two predominantly Muslim countries in the world today.

Next, I learned the price of freedom. I thought of all the immigrants to America who arrived at Ellis Island in times past, as well as other places that would take refugees around the world. What a road it was for each of them — gruesome at times. Many survived countless horrors in order to find the hope of freedom. Freedom is too often taken for granted. By me, by us all. Helping others to find freedom is the best way to recognize how precious it is.

Finally, I learned of our responsibility to others. I continually tried to answer the question of how I really felt about the crisis. Should countries be letting refugees in freely, as some did, or should they be more carefully screening or even turning away individuals seeking asylum? How did I feel about this as a Jew? As an Israeli? As an American? As a human being?

There are real and complex issues here, making simple solutions impossible. Our moral responsibility as human beings and as Jews to help refugees is clear but, at the same time, we would be irresponsible not to acknowledge the possible dangers that exist.

We must also be blind to cultural, ethnic, or racial differences. Humans help humans. Not long ago, in the Israeli Knesset, a right-wing orthodox member argued that Jewish doctors shouldn't have to treat an LGBTQ+ person and that they should be sent to non-Jewish doctors. That angers me.

An overlooked issue is how refugees inevitably deal with mental health issues, even if they didn't suffer from them before they were displaced. Anxiety, stress, insomnia, depression — these can be brought on by traumas. The world is barely able to look after refugees from a physical standpoint — feeding, housing, caring for bodily injury. The mental health plight has barely been examined, and yet it can be just as devastating. It was traumatic for me to see the refugees while voluntarily there to assist them in any way I could. It's possible that my volunteer work has negatively affected my psyche, but that's a risk I've been willing to take because my problems are so minor compared to those of the people I hope I've helped.

I travel to help others, but also to help myself. Perhaps "help" is the wrong word. I travel to challenge myself, to learn, to confront, to open up new pathways that wind through my mind. There's a self-serving element to any selfless act and, for me, the act of helping refugees was also about helping me learn more about myself.

Talking about facts and figures is often much easier than talking about our own attitudes, beliefs, and feelings. But I will say that, while I learned a great deal of facts, most of what I learned challenged my heart as much, or more, than my head.

As I think back on the volunteer experience as a whole, I begin by acknowledging that it was emotionally tiring, challenging, downright draining. However, it was also an incomparable experience to provide succor to someone from whom you neither want nor expect thanks. Service without expectation of reward is a beautiful thing.

Volunteer service reminds me of how truly amazing we humans are, of how pure we can be at the core. We are capable of coming together, regardless of race, nationality, or religion, despite any obstacle, despite any emotions. In Greece, when I saw that someone needed assistance, I jumped right in, with a smile on my face, and even my own dry sense of humor.

My journey to Greece was just a short plane ride away. The time and cost for the refugees who made their journey were so much greater. A commercial ferry ride from Turkey to Greece costs around $20. But the "non-commercial" route, can include payments to smugglers, which brings the cost up to some $1,500 per refugee. That doesn't even mention the costs to body and spirit — the long trudges from country to country, the dangerous boat rides, the individuals lost to the sea or sniper bullets. Their stories remind me of the nature of true courage.

After my volunteer time ended, I asked myself: where do we go from here? The refugee "solution" is not a simple one, as evidenced by all the controversy that surrounds the situation and every new iteration of it, more recently with the Ukraine war. It takes us all out of our comfort zones.

Most of us hang out in our own little worlds — mine is Judaism, Zionism, dealing for the most part with people who share our habits, beliefs, and attitudes. I know that I spend at least 90% of my own time with people who share a love of Judaism and/or a love of Israel. On Facebook, most groups I belong to are the same. I get "likes" from my friends and sometimes from their friends who are part of the same (at this point voluntary) "ghetto." Like many, I seem to prefer an echo chamber that affirms my own opinions. Yes, I like to have my opinions liked.

I think of this social media phenomenon when I think about the refugee situation. As much as, idealistically, I would love to accept the refugees I met into Israel, I know that for many reasons it's impractical if not impossible. What would the reactions of those I helped have been, had they known that I wasn't just an American — which for some might have been bad enough — but a Jew ... and an Israeli? I like to think that there would have been no negative reaction at all. After all, I was a human helping another human and asking nothing in return. But I didn't want to find out. I preferred to not poke the dormant beast in the room, to live on the level of humans to humans. I really couldn't hide being American — inevitably conversations shifted to where we were from, and my American voice would've given me away. I chose to volunteer as an American but neither Jewish nor Israeli. That's a shame that I felt the need to hide what is really the most significant part of my identity.

Since Israel isn't an option, I found myself wishing I had an "in" and an influence on those in the twenty-two Arab countries that might take in their neighbors. For seventy years, the Arab countries have not accepted even Palestinian refugees, whereas Israel is a country almost entirely populated by refugees. Many of them came from Arab or other Muslim countries.

Originally, I had very mixed feelings about letting refugees into others' countries. But after my week volunteering, I would encourage anyone who holds negative views about refugees to go out — from wherever they may reside — and interact with them. That may be the last thing that someone prejudiced against refugees would want to do, but it's what they *should* do. The Syrian people are not the terrorists. The refugees are not the terrorists. They are fleeing from those who are.

I see both sides of the coin on this topic and certainly understand the fear. I don't claim to have the ideal solution in mind. At one point I read that Canada was welcoming 25,000 Syrian refugees. Canada is my next-door neighbor. What happens in the future if just one of these immigrants is involved in a terrorist act? On the other hand, do you condemn 24,999 individuals for the possible actions of one? I've concluded that, with proper vetting procedures (not yet in place), I'm willing to take the chance.

I learned that most refugees are educated, kind, and calm. I was humbled to see their reactions to these awful situations and how, at their core, they are peaceful. I couldn't say the same about myself in such a situation. And I learned that we all have moral obligations to which we must adhere.

What are these obligations? What are *my* obligations?

My primary obligation: not to remain silent. I can't pretend that this situation and others like it aren't happening. I have no intention of screaming from the Temple Mount or blasting social media with my thoughts. But I do plan to share my learning and findings with anyone who is interested in hearing them — anyone who is willing to step outside of our little voluntary ghettos for even a few minutes. It's not all just a bad dream. While these refugee situations are not comparable to the Holocaust, we must be aware that there are some groups such as the Yazidis, Kurds, and various Middle Eastern Christian groups, like the Chaldeans, who are even now being targeted for mass murder. How can we help them? Let us not forget the righteous gentiles who helped the Jews. As a righteous Jew, do I not have an obligation to do likewise?

As a *Jew*, I have an obligation to help because it is what I've been taught to do and what I've taught my children. It is what I try to set as an example for my fellow citizens of whatever race or religion.

As an *Israeli*, I have an obligation to help because, while we continue to (and should) look out for ourselves, we must not forget others, as we have been taught.

As an *American*, I have an obligation to help because much of my family arrived on the shores of the United States and were taken in as refugees, and for that reason, I am here. While we need to be vigilant, we need to remember that we can do so in a humane manner.

As a human being, I have an obligation to help because that is part of what makes us human. I can hope that anyone reading this will feel the same. Help can be in whatever form or manner with which each of us is comfortable.

I learned all this through travel. Not for fun, not for a holiday, not to unwind. Travel to help others. Travel to find an uncharted piece of myself.

This is what I strive to live by.

This is what I learned.

This is what was reinforced during my week helping refugees in Greece.

I cannot just sit here and pretend it's not my problem.

I hope you can't, either.

Chapter 18

Therapy is a Journey

You

Even a happy life cannot be without a measure of darkness, and the word happy would lose its meaning if it were not balanced by sadness.

— Carl Jung

While I love a deal (remember all those Gonzaga sweatshirts), I go all-in and pay whatever it takes when it comes to healthcare for me and my family. When I realized that, where I now live in Israel, there is little to none of the diversity of mental healthcare options available in the US, I made it a project to bring these possibilities to Israel. This is not just for me but as a legacy for my country.

I've experimented with a vast array of therapies — traditional, alternative, and "out there" — to heal myself. For the ultimate round-the-world journey ends where it all began: within ourselves. Travel has taught me this: there is no enemy but ourselves. Back when Dafna was in treatment in the US, Israel had compulsory military service, but women could choose between serving in the army or in the National Service. Dafna opted for the latter, a two-year commitment. The first year she was at home in Israel, helping children with special needs. For the second year, she was asked to go abroad. She went to Houston, to work with local youth there and give them a flavor of Israel — a sort of public relations ambassador.

A short while into her time there she let us know that she wasn't happy. It didn't make sense to me or Carol, because this had been a dream of hers. Looking back at the Hurricane Sandy relief trip, Dafna had loved the role of informal ambassador of Israel to young Americans. At the time, neither Carol nor I were in tune with mental health issues. I'd been in therapy, but so have one in six Americans, according to a 2004 study, and I'd not yet delved deeply because I hadn't yet realized the extent of my own problems. We had no idea that Dafna was suffering. We imagined it was just homesickness or something minor.

A few weeks into her time in Houston, Ilan got married. The wedding was in Toronto, and we all flew to be there, Dafna, too. Dafna was so happy to be with the family but was crying about having to go back to Houston. Again, we figured she was homesick. Our other kids were more in tune than Carol and I were. Dafna did go back to Houston and, after a few weeks, our other kids grew concerned. We spoke and all decided she should come home. This was when we recognized that she was suffering and she began her therapy, which continues to this day.

I resumed therapy myself back in the midst of the pandemic, in 2021. That, too, felt like a situation in which external factors were making things harder for me — concern for Dafna and the lockdown, which was hard on so many. I felt good with the original therapist but also felt that I wanted to try more approaches and see if therapy with others would be different and helpful in new ways.

That was when I began my aforementioned therapy experiment, auditioning many approaches and doctors. My initial focus was on trauma. I started to work with two different trauma therapists at the same time, working different modalities.

Dafna's Israeli therapist was trained in Dialectical Behavioral Therapy. DBT is good for those who experience emotions so intensely that it can be debilitating. It's based on Cognitive Behavioral Therapy but involves more of a taking approach and focuses on how thoughts can affect emotions, and emotions lead to behaviors. A counterproductive thought-emotion-behavior loop can be broken by the right therapy. An example of a productive version of this loop might be a) thought: I'm not good enough at math; b) emotion: I feel badly about this, so; c) behavior: I'll study harder until I get my grades up. A destructive version of the same loop might be a) thought: I'm not good enough at math; b) emotion: which I extrapolate to feel that I'm not good at anything and I'm a worthless person so; c) I want to self-harm or drink or do drugs because I feel so badly about myself.

Dafna was learning new skills; techniques that she might apply to help herself in the future. I have a similar thought process when "harvesting" therapy techniques — I figure the more I'm exposed to, the better I'm equipped to help myself with some combination of them. I feel it's leaving it too much to fate or luck to hope that the first therapy approach you're exposed to will be the one that sorts you out.

More important than the specific approach is finding a therapist who feels right for you. This is not necessarily a judgment call on the objective quality of the therapist in question. Someone just right for one person might not feel good to another patient, and vice versa. It's also about timing — at one stage a therapist might be helpful but at another stage in one's mental wellbeing journey another therapist might be preferable.

This is all to say that walking you through my own therapy journey, or Dafna's, isn't likely to be helpful or particularly enlightening. What may be useful is this unusual approach of mine, the harvesting of self-healing techniques from a wide array of therapy modalities. That's a strategy I've not heard others preach and I think it's a good one.

That's the journey part of it.

Finding "the perfect" therapy or therapist would be a quest, a destination-driven journey. What I'm suggesting is that the journey itself is the point. Travel through different ways to heal yourself. Gather what seems useful as you go. You'll end up with a virtual backpack full of techniques that are tools that you can use to self-heal. It's you who heal your own mental sufferings in the end. The therapist is just there to guide, encourage, suggest, and equip you with techniques.

I don't think Israir started my issues. I think it triggered what I now feel was present all along. I didn't know it was there before, but now I think that it was. And though I still have trouble accepting it, I think this all began with childhood trauma. There have been triggers along the way: Israir, Dafna's illness, and the pandemic — which affected many around the world. When Dafna began her mental wellness journey, I reflected on my own. There was an overlap, but it was not a direct cause and effect.

There were smaller triggers, as well, that have led me to explore "betrayal trauma" incidents in which I felt in some way betrayed by an institution, or rather individuals within them, that were important to me. Some have a single traumatic incident. That can be more straightforward to soothe.

My experience is a mosaic.

Perhaps yours is, too.

But mine is also a journey that I do not expect to end definitively.

One of the techniques I learned from ACT therapy is the idea that it's easier to accept a mental wellbeing issue as a part of me that I should learn to live with. I can learn to live *around* it, wrapping it in cognitive techniques that render it as non-intrusive and innocuous as possible. But that's an easier goal than attempting to excavate, extract and destroy it altogether. After all, it is a part of me. Let the mental wellness journey be an endless wrapping in gauze, making the aspect of my mind that causes me discomfort nonmalignant.

Living with it might be an act of self-compassion.

Having now told several stories among my numerous volunteer journeys around the globe, I find myself considering why I'm so drawn to volunteer work. My therapist(s) would probably say that it is my method of sublimating the pervasive sense of guilt that flows through my veins alongside all those red blood cells. Why guilt when I've not done anything objectively objectionable? I don't have a grandfather who was in the SS, like Olaf the tour guide in Germany, so I don't even know of a story of an ancestor I whose behalf I feel I should atone.

I've always been drawn, without knowing why, to help total strangers in the worst of times. Perhaps it's my inner Judaism emerging in the form of beneficial projection. It's hard to find a community more hard-done-by than the Jews, dating back as many millennia as you like. Maybe I try to embody the sort of person I wish had been there to help my people over the centuries.

Is that enough of a reason to leave my family behind (although some of them would have liked to be here as well)? To abandon my work responsibilities and travel 10,000 kilometers, at my own expense and without a real plan in tow? Is insane, irresponsible (to myself) humanitarianism a thing? No doubt I was doing good, however minor my actions were in the grand scheme of things. I just had this inner feeling saying, "Do it."

Some might describe that inner feeling saying, "Do it," as the voice of G-d. It's why Abraham was ready to sacrifice Isaac (to pick a less sunshine-y example), and why Noah built an ark. Therapists tend to avoid the will-of-G-d explanation and go with the will-of-guilt.

Guilt can be a powerful force of good. Much philanthropy stems from the inner monologue: "I have a lot. Others have too little. Let me give some of what I have to those who have less." Instead of sending money, I "send" myself.

Perhaps the key aspect of psychotherapy is the shift, often ever so slight, in perspective, from seeing a situation in your life as problematic and negative, and realizing that, when viewed from a different angle, the same situation unaltered, appears positive, or at least no longer problematic.

This is the teaching of David Burns, the multi-million best-selling psychiatrist who authored *Feeling Good*. One of his examples is from a patient who felt terrible about herself, even suicidal, because she was always at work and didn't feel she had spent enough time with her children when they were younger. Regret ate at her. But Burns helped her shift the viewpoint of the exact same situation. Why did she work so hard? To give her family the best possible quality of life, sending her kids to schools where they could thrive, ensuring they wanted for nothing. So she was working hard as an expression of her love. And did her children feel they missed out? No, she said, they never did, it's just the way I see it when I look back. So the new interpretation of the same situation is spun positive: the woman worked hard as a show of love, for the benefit of her children. She was doing what, at the time, she thought was right. It turned out that her kids thought it was right, too. It was only after she retired that she interpreted her life with regret.

As I have said to my kids since infancy: "Do what you think is right." Although I was never sure of what the right answer is, and exactly what impact my actions may have (on others or on me), I've always opted to listen to myself and to do what I think is right.

This is what really brought me to the Philippines, the land of 7,107 islands.

Is it necessary to travel so far to feel a sense of self-worth? Recall my work dysmorphia — no matter how much work I do, I'll still perceive that it isn't enough. My travel and my volunteering and my travel to volunteer are beneficial for those I help, but examples of my compulsive behavior fueled by dysmorphia, a preoccupation with doing work in general, with doing good deeds as but one manifestation of it. But if I traveled a thousand miles, or ten thousand, if I helped one person or one hundred, I would still perceive that I could have, and should have, done more. It's the "should have" that gets you. If it were just about "could have" then maybe I could shrug it off. But "should have" implies compulsion, regret, guilt at having not done enough, which is followed by determination to do more next time. That my focus is volunteer work means that there are positives emerging from my compulsion, but it doesn't make it easier on me. I feel great when I'm helping people but as soon as the moment passes, I feel a pressurized void within me that urges me to do more. I'm facing my problems outward, looking for external things — places to go, people to help — to soothe my inner turmoil. But no matter how much I do, I'm still stuck with the turmoil, because it's within me.

That's what this book really is about. As I was writing it, I was sure I could avoid the cliché of the journey in search of one's self may cross a hundred borders, but in the end, you find that the answer is within you. Well, I suppose cliches are there for a reason. I think the answer is not as clean as to say, "Don't bother traveling the world to find yourself. Just stay put and look within." That may work for some (with a good therapist as your "wingman"), but for me, I found the literal journey to be a hugely helpful, necessary step to finally breaching the borders of my own self. I wouldn't have been able to find the answer within without all that actual travel around the globe.

Not that I've found the answer within, not definitively. That's also too clean and brings me to the next extension of my analogy, and very true cliché number two: The journey is the point, not the destination. With mental health and emotional wellbeing, there isn't a destination. You may think there is. If I buy this car, I'll be happy. If I get this job, I'll feel good about myself. I just need to get married. Have kids. Buy a house. Buy a weekend house. Buy a car. No, another car, the fast one with too little space in the trunk. Play the Saint Andrews golf course. Snorkel with sharks on the Great Barrier Reef. Climb Mount Everest.

Those are all wonderful experiences, but we can't expect the experience alone (let alone a purchase) to be the key to the lock within us, behind which lies happiness. Though I'm a devout Jew, the Buddhists are onto something. Desire is often the problem. Desire for what we don't have, that blinds us to what we do. Maybe happiness, or at least contentment, is the absence of desires beyond one's reach. Take the journey, enjoy the journey. The journey should be a blessing in itself, regardless of whether or not you reach — or even have — a destination.

My life has been a series of journeys, literally and metaphorically. I see my own mental health as a journey, as well. That has helped. At first, I was looking for the one big fix. The ah-ha therapy breakthrough that would suddenly heal it all. As in: we uncover from my subconscious that my mother did X on my birthday and since then I've felt Y, which I internalized, and it's led me to the diagnosis of living with psychological burden Z. It doesn't work like that, neither life nor therapy. The journey is a series of discoveries, about the world around you and about yourself.

Never stop journeying.

EPILOGUE

Lost. That's what I often feel. While this is the confession of a non-traveler when he finds himself in a new place, it could just as well be the confession of someone traveling the road toward mental health. This road can feel lonely, but it needn't be. While the minutiae, the details of our stories, trials, pasts, feelings compose a unique mosaic for us all, the journey of mental wellbeing is a ubiquitous aspect of the human condition. We all have good days and bad, optimistic days and challenging ones, moments of anguish and euphoria, times of blues and bright bursts of ecstasy. We are all on this path together, even if we can feel very alone at any given moment. We need reminders that we are not lonely travelers. That's why we need more Stuart Katzs. We need more people sharing their stories. The statistics in the DSM won't teach us that we are not alone. The voices of real people will.

Stuart Katz is a leader at the forefront of a mental health advocacy movement that is changing the way we think about, talk about, and address mental health. His particular voice adds fresh and much-needed honesty and humanity to the conversation. Stuart is a person of incredible integrity, commitment, and grit, and I have witnessed the countless lives he has touched, and yes even saved – both directly and indirectly – through his tireless, often heroic, efforts. His stated goal with publishing this book is to save one life. He has already saved countless.

As a rabbi and a psychotherapist, I have had the privilege of walking alongside individuals from all walks of life, witnessing their joys, sorrows, and everything in between. I have seen firsthand that every person is on a unique mental health journey, a path that we all must navigate with compassion and understanding.

Just as physical health varies from person to person, so does mental health. Each individual carries within them their own mosaic of emotions, thoughts, and experiences that shape their mental well-being. We all face our own battles, past or future, known or still veiled, and it is important to remember that we cannot fully comprehend the struggles of another.

The journey of mental health is not linear. It is a continuous process of self-discovery, healing, and growth, and it is inevitably waylaid by setbacks. Just as our bodies require care and attention, so too do our minds and spirits.

We must cultivate practices that promote mental well-being, such as prayer, mindfulness, and participation in supportive community. It is essential that we create contexts where people feel comfortable sharing their stories, seeking help, and finding solace in the embrace of a compassionate community. When someone opens themselves up, presenting their story, as Stuart does in this book, he has created a refuge where readers can meet a sympathetic, informed, compassionate soul halfway.

Mental health is not a solitary journey. It is a collective endeavor that requires us to extend a helping hand to those in need, to listen carefully and without judgment, and to offer support and resources. May we create a world where mental health is prioritized, stigma is dismantled, and every individual is given the space and opportunity to flourish on their own unique path towards well-being.

Interweaving a personal passion of his from outside of the mental health profession with a well-crafted narrative of his own mental health journey, Stuart has shown that mental health advocacy and mental health generally are best pursued in the larger context of what makes us each unique and, simultaneously what combines and connects us as humans. Stuart's style, combining humor, irony, and passion, make him an invaluable voice of demand for change – in the way we think about, prioritize, and address mental health in our ever more complicated world.

— **Rabbi Dr. Yehuda Septimus**

ACKNOWLEDGMENTS

I would like to express my deepest gratitude to all those who have played a significant role in making this book a reality. Your support, encouragement, and contributions have been invaluable throughout this journey.

First and foremost, I want to extend my heartfelt appreciation to my wife, Carol. Your steadfast love, understanding, and unwavering belief in me have been the driving force behind the completion of not only this book, but of me making it to this day. Your constant presence, patience, and support have been my anchor, inspiring me to persevere through the challenges of life and embrace the joys of writing.

To my children, Adina, Ilan, Gilad, and Dafna for your written contributions and together with your spouses and children – Ophir, Margalit, Naomi, Lielle, Eitan and Ayelet - thank you for your understanding and patience during the countless hours I spent immersed in this project and so many others. Your enthusiasm, creative insights, and steady belief in my abilities have provided me with the motivation and inspiration to bring this book to fruition. Your contributions, both big and small, have enriched the narrative and made it a truly collaborative effort.

To Adina, for creating the cover concept, and to Urška Charney, for seeing it come to life.

I would also like to extend my heartfelt appreciation to my family and friends, including Rabbi Yehuda Septimus, Rabbi Shmuley Boteach, Dr. Blaise Aguirre, Zak Williams, Tamir Goodman, Michael Sweetney, Reggie Williams, Brian Cuban, Asher Gottesman, Joshua Rivedal and Eric Kussin, who have supported me throughout this writing journey. Your words of encouragement, thoughtful discussions, endorsements, and constructive feedback have played a vital role in shaping the ideas and concepts explored within these pages. Your belief in me has been a constant source of strength. A special thank you to my dear friend, Gassen Alhoro, who showed me true resilience in the toughest of times and is a true model. And finally, to my dear friend Kevin Hines, for writing the Foreword and emphasizing the value of each day of life.

A special mention goes to Noah Charney, whose expertise and guidance have been instrumental in refining the content of this book. Your thoughtful insights, meticulous editing, and constructive criticism have elevated the manuscript to new heights. I am deeply grateful for your dedication and professionalism.

I would like to extend my gratitude to the publishing team at 3rd Coast Books for your belief in the potential of this book and your support throughout the publication process. Your professionalism, attention to detail, and commitment to excellence are deeply appreciated.

Lastly, I want to express my gratitude to all the readers and supporters who have embraced my work. Your interest, feedback, and words of encouragement have been a constant source of motivation. I am humbled and honored to have the opportunity to share my thoughts and experiences with you. As so many have asked, my goal in writing this book is this: I hope it can save just one life and give hope to all when hope is most needed.

This book would not have been possible without the love, support, and contributions of the remarkable individuals mentioned above. I am forever grateful for your presence in my life and for the role you have played in making this book a reality.

With deepest appreciation,
Stuart

ABOUT THE AUTHOR

Born in Panama, Stuart Katz is the epitome of a global adventurer. With his infectious wit and insatiable wanderlust, he has become a prominent figure in the world of travel. Leading a long-standing boutique travel company and having overseen the North American wing of Israir, he's the go-to guy for unforgettable adventures and witty recommendations. Stuart's op-eds and blogs have graced the pages of many publications worldwide, but this book marks his debut as an author. Alongside his travels to over one hundred countries, he's become a vocal advocate for mental health, spreading education, advocacy, and acceptance wherever he goes. If you enjoyed this book, you might also enjoy Stuart's podcast, also called Travel Therapy, and available where podcasts are found.

www.ingramcontent.com/pod-product-compliance
Lightning Source LLC
Chambersburg PA
CBHW030150100526
44592CB00009B/200